The Totally Wired Doctor

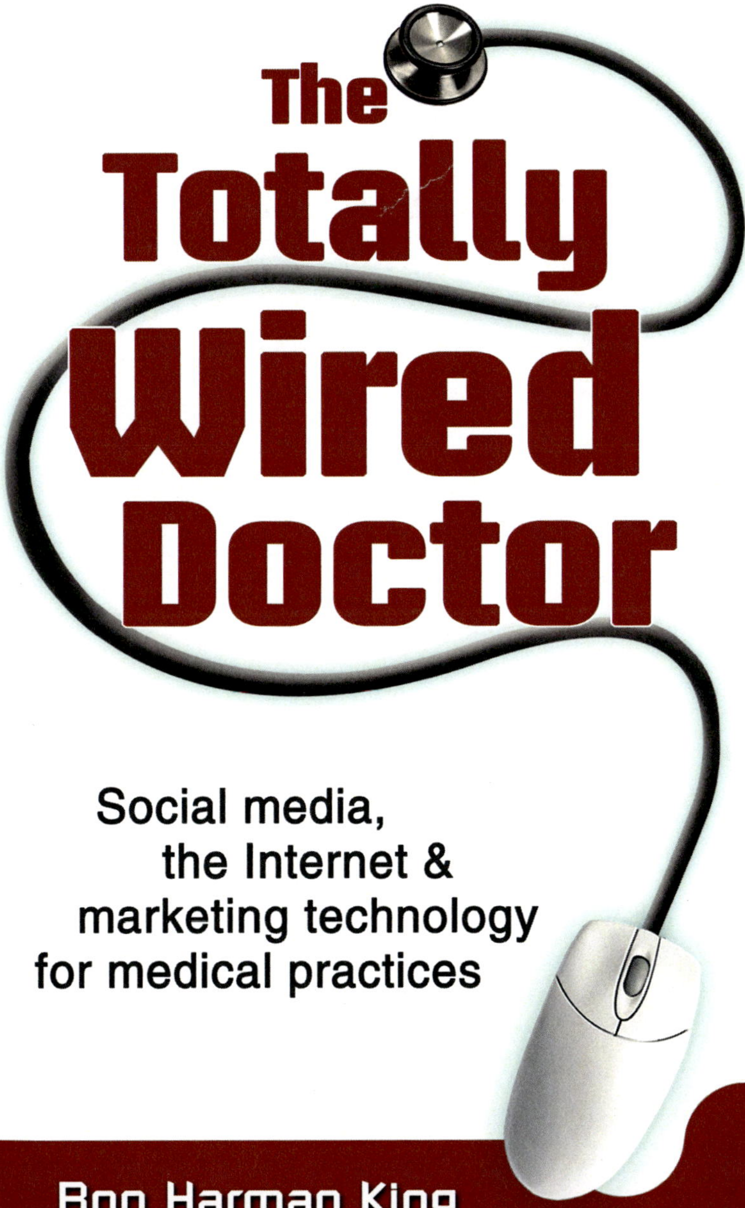

Social media, the Internet & marketing technology for medical practices

Ron Harman King
CEO, MedMarketLink

The Totally Wired Doctor:
Social media, the Internet & marketing technology for medical practices

Published by
Vanguard Communications
2400 Broadway, Suite 3
Denver, CO 80205

http://vanguardcommunications.net

For information about Vanguard Communications or its services, please visit http://vanguardcommunications.net or call 303-382-2999.

Table of Contents

About the author

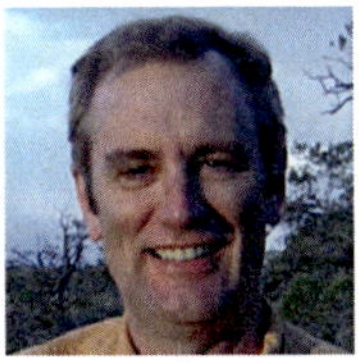

Ron Harman King is founder and CEO of Vanguard Communications, a Denver-based marketing, public relations and technology firm specializing in growing specialty medical practices and hospitals.

Since launching the medically-focused MedMarketLink program in 1998, Vanguard has combined the disciplines of online and offline PR, strategic marketing and information technology to bring new patients to physician specialists in fertility, neurosurgery, urology, orthopedics, oncology and dermatology from coast to coast. Ron is a recognized authority in the field of marketing and PR, appearing weekly as a commentator on KTVD/KUSA-TV 9 News, Denver's NBC affiliate.

During his graduate studies in information technology at the University of Denver, Ron analyzed how patients find and evaluate doctors and treatment options in the information age. He concluded that not just the Internet but also cable TV has upended the practice of medicine in less than 10 years: Whereas physicians once held the monopoly on health care knowledge, today patients increasingly mine the latest in medical research and news to control their own care and destiny.

Ron holds degrees from three universities in journalism, engineering and information and communications technology, as well as a certificate in French studies from the University of Lausanne in Switzerland.

For more information: http://vanguardcommunications.net

Who this book is for

1. Physician shareholders in private medical practices

2. Managers and administrators of medical practices with fiduciary, marketing and/or information technology responsibilities

My hat is off and my heart is out to the above. As will be noted repeatedly throughout this book, health care providers and executives are facing financial and operational pressures from all directions. This book is intended to help ease such pressures.

This work explores the formidable assortment of forces at play in determining the success of a medical practice. Health providers need a steady flow of new patients. Specialists need them even more than primary care providers. How and where do they get them?

Please note that this book is not for most technology professionals, especially those not interested in how the Internet affects health care consumer behavior.

Along with a comprehensive review of Internet-centered technology, the following pages review many of the elements of medical marketing and how patients select health care providers.

In short, we're turning the tables to talk about how patients examine doctors.

Foreword

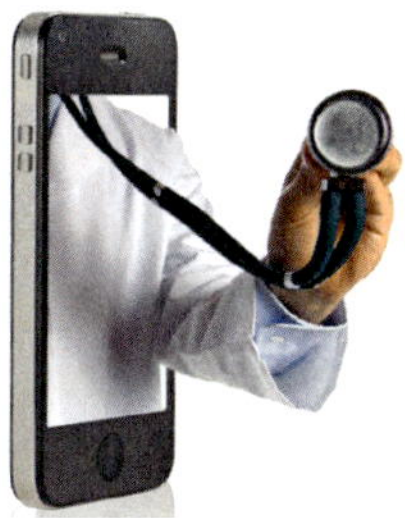

How connective technology upended health care

The best way to start this book is with a warning: reading it will not be worth everyone's time.

These days there are two kinds of medical practices – those that can live almost purely off referrals from other physicians (often primary care doctors), and those dependent on additional sources of new patients for practice success.

If you're part of a practice that falls in the first group, you can stop reading immediately and go do something else, something fun. Okay? Good, count yourselves lucky, even if only temporarily. Go enjoy that round of golf or time with your kids. See ya 'round.

For everyone else – you in the latter group dependent on a mix of new-patient sources – let's get down to business. Some of the others will be back to join our circle before long.

Just about everything in the business of practicing medicine has changed in some way in only two decades. Lofty visions of new and more cost-effective managed care programs have come and gone, and then something happened called the Internet. All the gargantuan changes in the American health care system have combined with the rise of new media to shift more and more power to health consumers.

Simultaneously, new regulations have curbed the advertising and marketing efforts of pharmaceutical companies, while declining reimbursements from payers have forced doctors to work harder and see more patients just to keep their heads above water.

My own primary care physician ruminated on this topic recently: "In 10 years, my practice expenses have risen 20 percent, while reimbursements from payers have dropped an average of 20 percent. The net effect is that I have to see 40 percent more patients just to keep the income I had 10 years ago."

Bottom line, physicians are being squeezed from all directions. Those who work for themselves can either sell their practices and become corporate employees, or they can do what the pharmaceutical and medical device companies started doing in the last century – talk directly to the health care consumer.

Where are the doctors in Consumer Reports?

Unlike previous generations, the 21st century patient won't settle for blindly taking instructions from physicians. The huge majority wants to be in control of their care and call the shots, starting with deciding which doctors they visit and whose advice they take.

How do patients pick doctors? What makes them stick with their choices? More and more, the processes are like the purchase of products such as computers, automobiles, televisions or even lawn mowers – but are still unique in many ways.

The wonderful news is that the best doctor-patient relationship will always be a close personal connection, and physicians will likely never have to hawk their services like car dealers shouting on TV commercials. (See Part II for more on this topic.) Sure, medical tourism seems to be drawing some patients to travel internationally for surgical procedures and other special care. Yet 95 percent of health remains a personalized and localized service for every patient. Even medical tourists are not likely to have more than one such experience in a lifetime.

The other wonderful news is that physicians who might feel a bit squeamish about the changing universe have the choice of avoiding that ugly M-word ("marketing") altogether. In health care, successful marketing lies far, far from the noisy end of the spectrum (i.e., obnoxious TV ads) and toward the most respectable end: patient education. Which brings us to a core principle in growing a medical practice:

Patients shop for information first & doctors second

In hopes of sorting through the hype of advertising, buyers of durable consumer goods frequently dive into objective reports and rankings online and in traditional media. The runaway popularity of websites such as Amazon.com (books, videos, music, etc.) and CNET.com (electronics and technology) is owed hugely to product and customer reviews. Consider:

Buyers of durable goods and services conduct from 60 to 80 percent of their research before initiating contact with sellers.

- Pew Research Center, 2012

Buyers want the unvarnished truth about sellers. Even in the Internet age when printed magazines seem to be going the way of dinosaurs, Consumer Reports magazine flourishes because of its hardball product evaluations and no-advertising-accepted publishing policy. Automotive shoppers in particular eagerly await the annual car-buyers-guide issue of CR each April with bated breath.

Health care consumers aren't so lucky. As of this writing, Consumer Reports – which meticulously examines how often last year's model of Toyota or Chevrolet winds up in the shop – has just begun a pilot project of making objective evaluations of physicians in the same manner.[1] The magazine's editors don't ever analyze a surgeon's performance by examining hundreds of his or her patient outcomes from, say, laparoscopic cholecystectomies (gall bladder removal). No can do.

When it comes to just how good a doctor is at his craft, patients are left with only two choices: 1) taking someone's word for it, either the doctor or some of the doctor's other patients, and 2) forming opinions on what they see and hear before, during and after visits to the doctors' offices.

An awful lot of these choices take place vicariously both in online and offline communications.

Medical marketing as a conversation

In short, it's all about trust. Selecting and sticking with a physician is largely a leap of... well, not exactly blind faith, but certainly sight-impaired faith.

The big trend in business these days is something called consumer-generated marketing. It's happening everywhere, including in health care. The basic concept is to have your best customers do a lot of the selling for you. And that starts with letting customers say just about anything about you they want, mainly on the Internet.

Customer-generated marketing was born out of the emergence of what's known as Web 2.0, the current ability to have two-way communications on the Internet. This feature, barely a few years old, reverses and upends a century of advertising and the tradition of talking about the seller first. It's the foundation of social media.

Similarly, patient-generated marketing is aimed at fostering conversation about the patient first and the doctor second. Picking a doctor is what professional marketers call a considered purchase, requiring the same careful consideration as buying a car or house or picking a school for your kids.

Shopping for many goods and services often begins with an Internet search, followed by browsing usually on several websites. This is the passive stage. With time, the shopper narrows her field of choices and begins the active stage: seeking information directly from a manufacturer, dealer or provider.

1 http://bit.ly/RcPsXU

In a comparable process, more than 8 million Americans go online every day to research health information, according to the Pew Research Center. But in contrast to other industries and professions, medical practices are woefully behind the Internet curve – astonishingly far behind, according to a report in Information Week magazine.

Citing a survey of nearly 5,300 patients by Forrester Research, IW concluded that "communication between physicians and patients via the Internet is still struggling to gain traction."

> Among so-called "e-Visit users" – patients who go online to communicate with their doctors – 46 percent have a college degree or higher. Among non-users, 25 percent have a college degree, barely half the rate.
>
> E-Visit users also have higher household incomes, averaging $88,000, while the average income for those not using the service is $70,000.
>
> Nine out of 10 e-Visit users said they go online every month and, when they do, they are more prone to conduct a variety of health research.
>
> Those who embrace the e-Visit experience also show greater signs of health care consumerism.
>
> A net effect of health care reform is that "the need for online conversations between doctors and patients will increase.

Based on this data, we draw several key conclusions:

> **Patients who use online communications with their providers are wealthier, more educated,** and are the most active regular Internet users and health consumers.
>
> **E-powered patients are better informed health care consumers with the best possible outcomes,** the very kind that practices should be pursuing as new patients.
>
> **Online health care communications are no longer the future but the present,** and individual medical practices have the choice of either leading or following their competitors.

Making the economic case

Okay, so the theory all sounds fine and dandy. Now come the brass tacks. Physicians and the medical world in general are particularly cause-and-effect oriented. Fittingly, the most common question about online communications and marketing for practices is, what evidence exists to prove that it's worth the time and cost?

I make a business case in the postscript at the end of the book. Feel free to skip ahead, read it, and then decide whether the words between here and there are worth your time.

Frankly, if you're involved in running a medical practice in a competitive environment, I'm certain that it is well worth your time.

In short, finding and recruiting new patients to a medical practice and converting the increased flow to business success usually require a persistent, multi-media, multi-resource and multi-disciplinary approach. This is not simple stuff. The average American receives hundreds of commercial messages a day – what makes your messages more captivating or relevant? The Internet contains an estimated 250 million to 350 million websites – how can you be so sure the right people are visiting yours?

This book is the distillation of 30-plus years experience in my career as a journalist, public relations and marketing consultant, and information technology professional. Here in these pages I've attempted to organize the decades of lessons into three buckets:

Part I summarizes the history of health care and the Internet, laying the foundation for why and how medical practices should adapt to the times, as well as an overview of how the Internet works (relevant for health care professionals).

Part II reviews medical marketing principles, which in large part are drawn from decades of successful marketing strategies and techniques for other consumer goods and services. While modern marketing is focused on the Internet medium, the time-tested principles of branding and targeted messages still apply.

Part III dives into the details of Internet marketing for medical practices, an attempt to untangle the complexities of social media, search engines, blogging and so on.

I hope to bring some clarity to the gamut of disciplines and topics intertwined in the modern marketing of medicine, as well as in health care management in general. This book is for those restless souls in search of providing not just better health care but also better health care information. This achievement, in my observation, is the fastest track to the next level of business success in medicine.

Leader or follower – which will your practice be?

Part I

What's happened to medicine in the 21st century?

Chapter 1

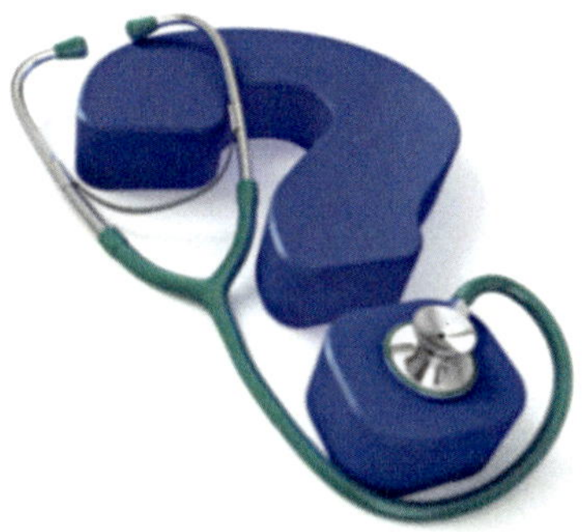

Who's in charge in health care today?

Hey, where did the gatekeepers go?

Imagine a world, if you will, in which you visit the local supermarket, select a grocery cartful of items sufficient to feed a family of four for a month, and at the cash register you pay $20 for a bill exceeding $300.

It's then up to the supermarket's management to collect the balance from a starvation insurance company, which has the obligation to its stockholders to reimburse the supermarket for as little as possible. In other words, the buyer sets the price. Or, rather, the buyer's all-powerful agent – typically a for-profit corporation and member of an industry cartel controlling billions of dollars in purchases – sets the price.

Outrageous? In any other industry, we'd likely never tolerate the system that we now know as American health care. For doctors, this system is only getting harder to tolerate, as fees for taking care of patients drop lower and lower while the cost of practice rises.

How did we get here? To arrive at its current state, the American health care system has traveled an extraordinarily winding road over the last century. The economic and social forces at play in medicine today took root long before passage of the Patient Protection and Affordable Care Act of 2010, and long before President Bill Clinton's reform attempts in the 1990s. Whereas the focus of 2010 reform was on requiring virtually all Americans to buy health insurance, Clinton's proposals were known largely for aiming to streamline costs through physician gatekeepers. Under the Clinton plan, patients' access to specialists would be limited to referrals from primary care doctors, thus reducing unnecessary and costly visits.

But gatekeepers are hardly new. In contrast to other industries, gatekeepers in one form or another have historically played some kind of role in the health care marketplace, a chaotic and convoluted mélange of buyers, sellers and third parties with various economic interests. The net result is a perpetual tug-of-war among groups with opposing interests.

And now, dear reader, it is time for a brief history re-cap. While this book is about using online media to build and sustain medical practices, remember that the Internet hardly exists in a vacuum. Really, the Internet is just a medium, like radio or television. In order to maximize its power, the savvy business owner/manager must place the medium in its proper context of the larger business universe. A bit of remedial review will help us arrive at an inescapable business-oriented conclusion (coming a little later in this chapter).

For the first 150 years of U.S. history, health care was haphazardly available, and health care insurance was practically non-existent. Doctors mostly treated sick people in their own homes and charged comparatively small fees or sometimes worked for free, since patients paid out of their own pockets.

By the 20th century, tonsillectomies, appendectomies and other surgeries had become common, and doctors were increasingly doing their work in hospitals. In the 1920s and '30s, medicine was undergoing rapid advancements, based in part on widening acceptance of the germ theory of disease and the emergence of antibiotics. As medicine took giant leaps forward in both preventing and managing disease, railroads became the first major industry to develop extensive employee health programs.

Industrialization spawns the rise of HMOs

In 1929, against growing industrialization, Dr. Michael Shadid enrolled several hundred rural families in the Oklahoma Farmers' Union. Members paid a set fee and received Dr. Shadid's care.[1] Shadid's initiative was born from a personal trait of humanitarianism as wide as the Oklahoma prairie. Having worked his way through Washington University in St. Louis by selling inexpensive jewelry door to door, Shadid had begun the practice of medicine by making rounds in rural Missouri and Oklahoma on horseback. In treating impoverished farmers' families, he found the widespread lack of health care appalling. As

1 http://bit.ly/Pa6QiQ

a consequence, he set out – at the onset of the Great Depression – on a lifelong crusade to overthrow the traditional fee-for-service practice dominated by solo practitioners.[2,3]

Historians today regard the formation of Shadid's farmers' union as the genesis of the health maintenance organization. However, his medical colleagues' initial reaction was less than joyous. The Beckman County Medical Society, where Shadid had been a member for 20 years, expelled him. The Oklahoma Board of Medical Examiners tried to revoke his license, and the State Medical Association lobbied the Oklahoma legislature to ban medical cooperatives.[4] But the determined doctor prevailed, and in 1931 he opened a cooperatively owned clinic and hospital in Elk City, Oklahoma.

Dr. Shadid was hardly alone in his quest for better, affordable care for the masses. Also in 1929, the Los Angeles Department of Water and Power contracted with two physicians to provide care for about 2,000 employees and their families.[5] A few years later, another group of Los Angeles physicians started serving 5,000 workers on an aqueduct construction project in return for a fixed monthly subscription fee, deducted from wages. Later, this same group did the same for construction workers on the Grand Coulee Dam for industrialist Henry J. Kaiser.

In the 1930s and '40s, prepaid group-practice plans proliferated. During World War II, Kaiser extended employee health services to workers in his shipyards and steel mills. Kaiser later opened his plans to the public, and eventually the Kaiser Permanente network became a dominant health care provider on the West Coast.

Popularity of HMOs grew to the extent that in 1971 President Nixon's administration announced a new strategy to make federal grants and loan guarantees to HMOs. On Dec. 29, 1973, Nixon signed the Health Care Maintenance Organization Act, legislation championed by Senator Ted Kennedy. The act required employers with 25 or more employees already offering traditional health care coverage to offer federally certified HMO options, too.

The appeal – and objective – of HMOs was to lower health care costs while simultaneously improving care outcomes by having primary care physicians deliver preventative care to patients through annual physicals, immunizations, mammograms, well-baby exams and similar efforts. Such care would catch and treat potentially serious illnesses and conditions before they became much more costly to address later. It would also help control the expense of managing such chronic diseases as diabetes, cancer and asthma.

2 http://to.pbs.org/QXVm29

3 http://bit.ly/Mmdo9J

4 http://bit.ly/NXro9Y

5 http://bit.ly/Pa6QiQ

Interest in wellness programs continued expanding in the 1980s as pressure to reduce unnecessary hospitalizations and boost efficiency increased for providers.[6] Concurrently, the nation shifted toward privatizing hospitals and health care.

Meanwhile, health insurers complained that health care providers were exploiting fees for services, and many moved toward capitation on payments, which meant paying doctors fixed annual amounts based upon the number of the insurance company's members who were in the doctor's care, regardless of individual treatment.[7] Medicare instituted other attempts at cost controls through the adoption of diagnosis-related groups, which in theory would place price controls on hospital services by classifying them into 467 groups.

Despite these measures, health care costs were rising at more than twice the rate of inflation by the 1990s. Ongoing attempts to rein in expenses sparked a consumer backlash. Customers began protesting that for-profit health insurers were more interested in cutting costs than improving care.[8] In addition, consumers became increasingly unhappy with the rigidity of HMOs, which generally limited choice in choosing hospitals and physicians.

In response, insurance companies drifted toward preferred provider organizations that allowed more consumer flexibility.[9] The trend from HMOs toward PPOs diluted hopes for doctor-gatekeeper benefits, as patients regained greater choice.

By the 21st century, modern economics and changing demographics led many industry leaders, politicians and academicians to believe that both Medicare and employer-based health insurance weren't sustainable. One proposed solution was to require more Americans to buy health insurance. This gave birth to the Affordable Health Care Act of 2010 – national legislation of enormous controversy. Following the Supreme Court's June 2012 decision upholding AHCA, health care professionals expect the new law has begun to revolutionize American health care.

Yet, another 20th century development is probably making a far greater impact on the health industry, not just in the United States but the world over.

The Internet ushers in the age of doctor shopping

Among the vicissitudes of American life, nothing in history has changed our decision-making behavior more dramatically than the advent of the Internet. In less than 20 years, the global computer network has become the indispensable companion of decision-making for every turning point in life. The Internet helps us decide where we work, live, and send our kids to school, and who we court and marry.

---

6 http://bit.ly/Pm8nk4

7 http://bit.ly/MGUdvC

8 http://bit.ly/Pm8nk4

9 http://bit.ly/MGUdvC

Given that the Internet is today's tool of choice for many of life's decisions, it's hardly surprising that health consumers consider their computers a vital health resource. Experts in this field certainly think so.

In a 2008 article in the Journal of the American Medical Informatics Association, George Demiris and others write: "Advances in information technology (IT) enable a fundamental redesign of health care processes based on the use and integration of electronic communication at all levels. New communication technologies can support a transition from institution centric to patient-centric applications."[10]

Patient-centric? You bet. In an Internet search for "loss of appetite," it takes Google just 0.08 seconds to sort and return 9.7 million Web pages. On a search for "child cough," it takes a mere 0.12 seconds for 49 million results to be returned. And it requires a scant 0.02 seconds more to get back 66 million results for "weight gain."

At latest count, there are more than 800 million Web pages on health topics. As expected, consumers have greeted instant access to a nearly infinite flow of health information with glee. The Pew Research Center in all probability has amassed the planet's largest repository of information on health care consumers' use of the Internet. According to the center's findings, 80 percent of Internet users and 59 percent of all Americans go online to learn about health. When you break it down by educational level, it gets even better: 89 percent of college graduates get health information online. Among Internet users suffering chronic health conditions, 83 percent depend on the Internet for health information.

Want to know what health care consumers are really interested in? Google will tell you all you care to know and a whole lot more. And it's free.

Because Google wants to sell advertising, it provides access to its colossal database of what search terms Google users select for information foraging on the Internet. (We cover this in more depth in Chapter 11.) The chart on the following page provides a few samples of the number of health-related searches conducted in Google each month.

The Internet explosion means that Americans make far more visits to health websites than they make to health care providers. It's difficult to over-estimate the impact on the medical profession. As any baby boomer can tell you, in a single generation, Americans have moved from nearly total dependency on doctor appointments (not just to get help for what's wrong with them, but also to find out what might be wrong with them), to having several ideas of the cause of their ailments – and possible treatments – in as little as eight one-hundredths of a second – all in the confines of their home or office cubicle.

---

10 Demiris, George and others, 2008. "Patient-Centered Applications: Use of Information Technology to Promote Disease Management and Wellness. A White Paper by the AMIA Knowledge in Motion Working Group." Journal of the American Medical Informatics Association, Vol. 15. No. 1, January/February 2008: 8-13.

Examples of monthly volume of Google searches, by keyword

hypertension	1.8 million
coughing	2.2 million
fertility	2.7 million
diarrhea	3.5 million
arthritis	4.1 million
physician	7.5 million
depression	9.1 million
weight loss	11.1 million
alcohol	20.4 million
diet	30.4 million
doctor	83.1 million

As much as PPOs weakened the control of doctor gatekeepers in the health care system, the Internet threatens to decimate primary care physicians' commanding influence over consumer selections of specialists and hospitals. Consumer-oriented websites that used to draw millions of visitors each month for movie, restaurant and hotel reviews are now raking in millions more with reviews of hospitals, medical practices and individual physicians. Shocking? Why should it be? Many couples won't even gamble $100 on a dinner out at a new restaurant before checking out its online reviews. Why would a patient facing knee replacement, back surgery or in vitro fertilization – all procedures costing tens of thousands of dollars – not first investigate the doctor's ratings among his or her prior patients?

Let us pause for a deep breath, and reflect on a common question: Are patient ratings of physicians a good thing? Well, patients certainly like them, as evidenced by the explosion of their popularity in just a few short years. Regardless of how doctors feel about them, online ratings are here to stay for most retail businesses – and I consciously include medical practices in that retail category.

At the same time, the Internet and free speech have their pluses and minuses in abundance. Since anybody can publish anything on the Internet, the proliferation of false and inaccurate electronic information is incalculable. This fact undeniably makes some patients sicker – and often annoys physicians – before they at last find efficacious care from skilled clinicians. Conversely, the cornucopia of accurate information has proven literally life saving for masses of patients and loved ones with discerning skills in assaying what they find online.

In any case, our task here is not to parse all arguments and render judgment on the goods and ills of new media, but rather to deliberate on our choices of response. We won't change or certainly turn back the Internet tsunami. We will only hope to respond to the massive wave constructively. It's sink or swim.

The medical establishment reacts

Let's look at who's in the biggest danger of sinking. What has been the response to the tsunami from the largest medical organization in the United States? Slow and stumbling at best – at least in the first 10 years of the Internet boom.

Not long ago, a search of The Journal of the American Medical Association (JAMA) website using the term "information technology" yielded a notable difference in tone and number of findings compared to the same search on the websites of the New England Journal of Medicine (NEJM) and the British Medical Journal (BMJ). In addition to fewer results, JAMA's website search returns articles that tend to have been published more than five years ago and represent a strongly cautionary view of the Internet. A sampling of article abstracts and conclusions express warnings such as:

"Despite its obvious benefits, the increase in the availability of [online health] information could also result in many potentially harmful effects on both consumers and health professionals who do not use it appropriately."[11]

"Accessing health information using search engines and simple search terms is not efficient. Coverage of key information on English- and Spanish-language Web sites is poor and inconsistent, although the accuracy of the information provided is generally good. High reading levels are required to comprehend Web-based health information."[12]

11 Jadad, Alejandro and Anna Gagliardi. 1998. Rating Health Information on the Internet. The Journal of the American Medical Association 279, No. 8: 611-614.

12 Berland, Gretchen and others. 2001. Health Information on the Internet: Accessibility, Quality, and Readability in English and Spanish. The Journal of the American Medical Association 285: 2612-2621.

"Who owns medical information? The one who gives care, receives care, or pays for care? All of the above? None of the above? Does it really matter? In the emerging era of electronic health information, few other medicolegal questions are more critical, more contested, or more poorly understood."[13]

To its strong credit, the JAMA's news website amednews.com provides an impressive array of articles on the Internet and information technology. Regardless, the medical establishment traditionally has been rightfully concerned about the inconsistent accuracy of online health information. Left to their own untrained biases, patients make poor decisions all the time. Yet information on the information highway is very much like information everywhere else. Some of it's good; some of it's terrible; and a lot is irrelevant and downright boring. So what?

Now that the Internet allows anyone to be a publisher, has the Internet increased or decreased the portion of reliable and useful medical information available to the public? Is it an improvement over any other kind of layperson information and hearsay? Is the Internet better or worse than patient gossip?

On balance, I respectfully submit that the Internet has increased access to accurate – and life saving – information to a nearly infinite dimension. Just one website, WebMD, attracts more than 60 million visits every month. It's time to give people some credit for discernment skills: Nearly every article of its 2.5 million pages is physician reviewed. WebMD is Exhibit One that people want accurate health information.

To be sure, hype abounds on the Internet around medical research and new drugs still in trial. New media ensure that the opportunity to be led astray by information providers with commercial or other nefarious intentions has never been greater. At the same time, the delivery of heretofore-inaccessible medical knowledge to health care consumers is unequivocally the greatest gift of the Internet.

Even if I'm wrong, the AMA and the medical profession at large have a simple choice: Get with this Internet thing or let the hucksters win with propaganda. Sink or swim.

Inescapable conclusion: buyers matter

At last we reach the deduction promised earlier in this chapter – the cosmos of all that has ever been in health care and forever will be, only more so. If the history of health shows us anything, it's this: Patients have a mind of their own and the power to exercise it.

Just as the Internet has fueled the so-called Arab spring and other citizen uprisings in the political sphere, the medium similarly has handed unprecedented power to consumers of all goods and services. As New York Times foreign affairs columnist Thomas L.

13 Hall, Mark A. and Kevin A. Schulman. 2009. Ownership of Medical Information. The Journal of the American Medical Association 301: 1282-1284.

Friedman observed in his 2005 book, The World Is Flat, buyers and sellers of products and services are now sourcing from all over the world and exploring new markets in developing countries.[14] And they're not the only ones; health care buyers – i.e., patients – also now shop citywide, statewide, nationwide and even worldwide for professionals to treat them.

None of this is to say that we'll soon be importing our annual physical exams from China or Indonesia or Vietnam. Health care is still and will always be overwhelmingly a locally delivered service, as Friedman notes is typically the case with professional services. But gone are the days when Americans dutifully did nearly everything their family doc told them. History proves repeatedly that health care is subject to free-market forces and that whenever the pendulum swings far enough from buyer influence, it will begin to swing back again.

"Medicine is a business"

Among those free-market forces is the hard reality that health care prices fluctuate constantly. Or, more accurately, what health care providers can charge and collect in fees is under constant pressure. In reality, the federal government is the nation's single largest health care customer: Medicare and Medicaid account for 30 percent of the money spent on care in the United States. Throw in other federal and state reimbursements to providers and the total rises to 46 cents of every dollar spent on health care by a combination of federal, state and local governments.[15]

So it's of no small concern to physicians when the federal government moves to cut Medicare payments. Since private insurers usually base their contracted reimbursements to doctors on Medicare rates, as go the feds so go UnitedHealth Group, Cigna, Blue Shield and the rest of for-profit insurance corporations.

Does any other industry suffer such a third-party chokehold? In health care, a few very powerful members of a cartel come very close to setting market pricing. The end consumer does not directly decide what s/he will and won't pay for the services – that's the decision of the cartel to which s/he typically pays a monthly subscription fee. Meanwhile, the seller (the doctor in private practice) who interacts with the end consumer (the patient) is forced to accept whatever the cartel offers. Sure, private medical practices can try negotiating with private payers on fees for their services. But good luck.

UnitedHealth Group et al isn't waiting on their phone calls. The smaller the practice, the weaker its negotiating muscle, leaving physicians in solo practice in the worst of positions.

---

14 Friedman, Thomas. The World Is Flat. New York: Farrar Straus & Giroux, 2005.

15 http://bit.ly/QXXRl4

"My frustration level is at a nine or 10 right now," San Antonio breast-cancer surgeon Kathryn Wagner told the Associated Press in a news story on pending Medicare cuts to specialists, published November 13, 2010,

"As a businessperson, I can't budget at all because I have no idea how much money is going to come in," Dr. Wagner said. "Medicine is a business. Private practice is a business."

Bravo, Dr. Wagner, for speaking the truth. A physician in private practice is really an independent businessperson first and a scientist second. Yes, the downer about being in business for yourself is that you can't control prices and revenues. That's life in the entrepreneurial aquarium and the top reason many private physicians are taking salaried jobs at hospitals or large groups, or selling their practices to hospital corporations.

Fortunately, physicians do have options. And some are unique to their profession.

As political and economic pressures force Medicare reimbursements downward, many physicians find themselves in the unenviable dilemma of whether to accept new Medicare patients. Under Medicare, doctors are rewarded not for good patient outcomes but for sheer volume – quantity over quality.

Yet physicians have one very clear option to find better-paying patients. It's an ugly truth that the best-funded patients are usually employed and covered by private health insurance. This is embodied in the term "payer mix," one of the great euphemisms in business today. All it means is that it's not usually a great idea to rely on just one kind of customer.

And why should we? It's not a good business idea. Even upscale automaker Mercedes-Benz sells some of their cars for less than $35,000. Similarly, the legendary piano maker Steinway imports grand pianos from China for a retail price of less than $20,000, in contrast to the $50,000 to $150,000 prices on its instruments handmade by unionized labor in New York City.

In both cases, the idea is brand capture – bring new customers into the door who otherwise couldn't afford the premium product. Meanwhile, keep and grow your share of premium customers by also selling the pricier products to those with larger wallets. This strategy amounts to Mercedes-Benz's and Steinway's versions of payer mix. Customer diversity is generally good for business health, regardless of your profession or industry.

In the health care sector, let's likewise call premium patients by their business name: premium customers. There are ways to recruit more premium customers to a business known as a private medical practice. Most industries have being doing just this for decades. It's called marketing – an uncomfortable word for many physicians.

The good news about marketing a private medical practice is that it's often easier and more cost-efficient than marketing most other consumer services. In fact, if there's any comfort for marketing-resistant health providers, it's that it's not so much about advertising as it is information and knowledge sharing.

Capturing the power of pull marketing

Back to the unique advantages of medical practice: Unlike needing an oil change for your car, when you need a surgeon, you need a surgeon right away. Health care consumers are inarguably the most motivated buyers on the planet. The car can go another thousand miles before an oil change, but a woman who has found a lump in her breast knows she has to take action NOW.

And what action does this woman typically take? She goes to the Internet to learn more. Not to find a doctor necessarily, at least not right away. But to explore her options beyond what her PCP may have told her in a 20- or 30-minute encounter in an exam room.

This is called pull marketing: answering the prospective customers who are asking for information. The phenomenon is the opposite of push marketing, in which a seller pushes a message at prospective buyers in hopes of good timing. Television commercials and billboards are examples of push marketing, and they have limited effectiveness in health care for sheer mathematical reasons – only a tiny sliver of the push-message audience seeing the TV ad or billboard needs a breast surgeon. (We cover this in more detail in Chapter 5.)

The good news for private-practice physicians ... or, rather, owners of independent health care businesses ... like Kathryn Wagner is that the higher a patient's educational level and income, the more likely the patient will be a painstakingly-informed health care consumer.

Generally, the highly educated (and better insured) patient will have high-speed Internet access, will spend more time surfing the Web for treatment options, and will be more likely to find a physician such as Dr. Wagner.

Why? Because Dr. Wagner is an active provider of not just health care but health care information. It's free, and it's right there on her patient-centric website: www.breastsurgerysa.com.

Dr. Wagner will likely succeed in the long run as a businesswoman for several reasons:

- She recognizes that private medicine is a business, making you more open to meeting consumer needs on their terms.
- Her website and information are easy to find on the Internet. To test this, simply Google "breast cancer surgeons San Antonio" or "breast cancer San Antonio." As of the time of this writing, the website appears on page one of the results for the first query and page two for the second.

- The quality of this information is very high, including topics such as "Breast Cancer Myths," "Breast Cancer Factoids" and "Reduce Your Risk."

- Dr. Wagner has admirably acknowledged that breast cancer is all about the patient, not about the provider. One telling sign: The URL, or web address, for the website doesn't contain her name. Rather, it's about the patient's needs.

Thus, a prospective premium customer can find Dr. Wagner easily and will likely form excellent first impressions of her. She is well-positioned for customer diversity.

Mind you, I'm not unsympathetic to vulnerabilities to politics and the free marketplace. Yet it's important to remember that the uncertainty of revenue is every business owner's cross to bear. The upside in health care is that the specialty-physician's customer pool is extraordinarily defined and driven. Premium customers are looking precisely for a professional like you, a doctor who cares as much about the patient's heart and mind as her response to surgery.

As we often say in marketing, that's the kind of brand that money can't buy. It's also pretty much what the rest of this book is about. Remember, it's sink or swim.

In the perpetual tug-of-war among sellers, buyers and gatekeepers (be they hospitals, referral physicians or health insurers), the buyers still have an unshakeable grip on the rope. And with patients having more pull and power of choice than ever, the Internet can throw you the biggest life buoy you could ever hope for.

Chapter 2

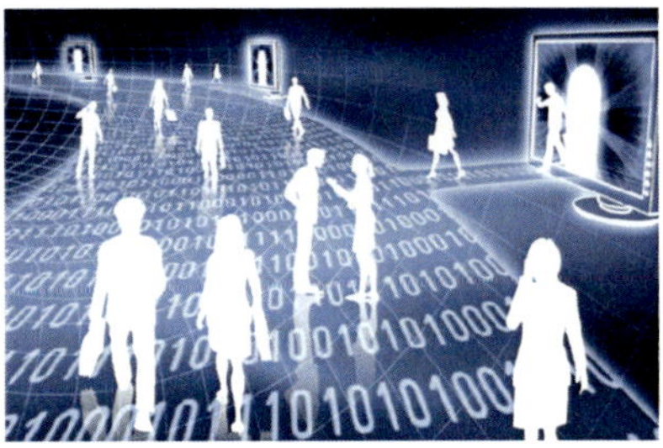

How the Internet works

& why health care professionals should care

The Internet's ubiquity – from Seinfeld to Bhutan

If we can thank anyone for reminding us how fast communications technology has changed, it's Jerry Seinfeld. Even after an unprecedentedly popular, nine-year run ending in 1998, the "Seinfeld" TV series continues to delight 21st century audiences the world over through syndicated re-runs, which show frequent glimpses of Jerry's then-state-of-the-art Mac II Apple desktop computer.

To appreciate both the growth and the reach of the Internet since Y2K (remember that antiquated term?), let us now go to a landlocked state in south Asia. A year after the production of "Seinfeld" ended, the Himalayan country of Bhutan lifted its longstanding ban on television and the Internet. In a 1999 speech to his countrymen announcing modernization initiatives, Bhutanese King Jigme Singye Wangcheck proclaimed television to be essential to national progress. (Some have speculated that the king's interest in TV rose principally due to "Seinfeld" going into syndication)

Today, Bhutan has roughly the same number of residents as Alaska (708,000 and 710,000, respectively), scattered across some of the tallest, most rugged mountains in the world. Four out of five Bhutanese are farmers, and annual per-capita income is a smidgen over $5,000, roughly one-eighth of Americans' earnings. Yet barely a decade after the end of the TV and Internet ban, broadband Internet access is available to subscribers in 48 locations nationwide.[1]

Bottom line, if you wanted to send a message halfway across the globe to a farmer working his rocky field in the Himalayas, you'd have decent odds of delivery via email. You might even have a better chance of getting back an email response from the farmer than from your primary care physician.

Origins: Another gift from Sputnik

Bhutan stands as stark evidence that the Internet has penetrated the farthest corners of planet Earth. Probably more surprising is the fact that the stunning reach of today's technology largely follows the 1961 vision of James Carl Robnett Licklider, a computer science professor at the Massachusetts Institute of Technology. Just four years earlier, the Soviet Union had launched its Sputnik satellite, setting off a Cold War technology race with the United States. Amid rising international tensions, scientists around the country scrambled to find ways to share research data quickly and securely.

In response, Licklider wrote a series of memos proposing an "Intergalactic Computer Network," a globally connected set of computers through which users could quickly access data and programs from any site.[2]

A year after his Intergalactic Network memos, Licklider was appointed as the first head of the computer research program at the Advanced Research Projects Agency (ARPA), established in 1958 within the U.S. Department of Defense. The mission of ARPA (which exists today as DARPA, for Defense Advanced Research Projects Agency) was and still is to head off any further Sputnik-style technology surprises by other countries.

By 1968, ARPA computer specialists had completed a plan for ARPANET, a computer network connecting defense researchers in multiple locations. The concept was considered so outlandish at the time that of 140 potential bidders who received an ARPA quote request for actually building the network, only 12 actually responded.[3]

The ARPANET contract eventually went to BBN Technologies who then went to work on the project's chief challenge, data flow. At this point in history, data transmission relied on circuit switching, which limited the ability to transmit data to one computer at a time.

BBN began expanding a different idea: packet switching, developed by an MIT scientist, Leonard Kleinrock. This allowed data to be broken into little bits and queued for distribution so they wouldn't clog the information pipeline. Although this would take place in

1 http://bit.ly/STZaAp

2 http://bit.ly/OZVJDt

3 http://bit.ly/QEwYTm

tiny fractions of seconds, speed was still a concern if hundreds or perhaps thousand of computers were to be linked together.

Another challenge that still exists today is that not everyone uses the same kind of computer using the same kind of operating system and software. Even if you delivered data to computers on the network, not every computer would be able to do anything with it.

To solve this puzzle, the ARPANET team began development of software called the Interface Message Processor. The IMP essentially became an independent minicomputer installed at each ARPA research site in order to translate data for local computers. The IMP remained in use until 1989, eventually morphing into what we know today as a router.[4]

Hence, the concurrent development of the IMP and packet switching would lay the foundation upon which the Internet still sits today, a half-century later. At the time, these technology pursuits did not go unnoticed by some important people, even in the earliest stages. In December 1968, Senator Ted Kennedy, grateful to see so much intellectual toil taking place in his state of Massachusetts, sent a somewhat confused telegram to BBN Technologies, congratulating the firm on winning the contract to develop the "interfaith message processor."[5]

In the fall of 1969, BBN installed the first IMPs at the Network Measurement Center at the University of California at Los Angeles and the Stanford Research Institute and subsequently sent the first message over the nascent network. One by one the ARPA team installed IMPs at other universities. By 1972, the ARPANET had connected 15 sites,[6] and in October of that year, its developers proudly gave the first public demonstration of the network at the International Computer Communication Conference.

The triumph of ARPANET (and its eventual descendent, the Internet) is owed to what's known as open architecture networking. In this approach, any work site – a research laboratory, office or private home housing an array of computers – can have its own local network that limits who has access. The site's computers can communicate within that local network regardless of each computer's operating system, and each computer can also communicate with virtually every other computer on the global network, a.k.a. the Internet. You get the best of both worlds.

Access to ARPANET took its next big leap in 1981, when the National Science Foundation created the Computer Science Network (CSNET). The purpose was to connect computer science departments at universities and research institutes that otherwise could not connect directly to ARPANET due to funding or authorization limitations.[7]

4 http://bit.ly/MHn6G6

5 http://bit.ly/NuW9r0

6 http://bit.ly/NJKEct

7 http://bit.ly/MWzvmm

The following year brought a related breakthrough. In 1982, the U.S. Department of Defense declared a new network protocol as its standard. In computers, a protocol is a system of defining rules and conventions for internetwork communications among computers. The first set of ARPANET conventions was the Network Control Protocol; by the mid-1980s, NCP was widely replaced by the Transmission Control Protocol and the Internet Protocol, or the TCP/IP.

The TCP/IP had been in development since the early 1970s by the so-called fathers of the Internet, Robert E. Kahn and Vinton Cerf.[8] (Kahn had also been involved in the development of packet switching.) TCP/IP simplified the network's job to merely transmitting and routing data. All other computing would be done at the so-called nodes of the network – by the computers themselves. This new approach allowed even more diverse computer systems to connect to ARPANET.[9]

Three decades later, TCP/IP still stands as the bedrock methodology of sending and receiving data packets over the Internet. (Remember that term "IP" for later; it's important for understanding search engines.) Kahn and Cerf went on to found the influential Internet Society in 1992, which has since grown to more than 50,000 members and sets much of the policy and direction for Internet development.

Further etching Kahn's and Cert's names into computing history, in 2005, President George W. Bush awarded the two pioneers with the Presidential Medal of Freedom. Today, Cerf is a Google employee with the title of Chief Internet Evangelist. Nice work (and name plaque) if you can get it.

A matter of conCERN to physicists & students

As providence would have it, one early adapter of the TCP/IP protocols in the 1980s was an international physics laboratory situated on the border of Switzerland and France. The Conseil Europeen pour la Recherche Nucleaire (European Council for Nuclear Research, later renamed), known as CERN, had been the 1952 creation of scientists from 12 countries wanting to collaborate on studies of nuclear physics. With hundreds of scientists, projects and computers under its umbrella, CERN needed a way to organize and track information about who was working on which project, as well as what affiliated software ran on which computers.

In 1990, two CERN scientists – Robert Caillau, a native of Belgium, and Tim Berners-Lee, an Englishman – persuaded their bosses to allow them to develop software connecting the laboratory's databases through text links on computer screens. The software they came up with possessed three interdependent components:

8 http://bit.ly/PmfaKJ

9 http://bit.ly/OirwmN

Hyper Text Transfer Protocol, which allows one computer (a "client") to submit a request for information from another computer (a "server"). This is the "http" you still see today in web addresses.

Hyper Text Markup Language, or HTML, a computer language that uses tags, or special annotations, to interpret and present documents to a Web browser in ways the browser can understand. (More on this below.)

The first Web browser, a software application for retrieving and presenting information on a computer monitor following the commands of HTML.

This trio of elements would completely transform human interaction with computers forever. The traditional display of dull text on a dark or white background could now morph into electronic pages with visual and audio functions. With these developments, by adding moving pictures, music and narration right there on a screen, a computer could present a better page than any book or magazine could. The CERN innovators decided to call their system the World Wide Web. The Web, as it soon became known, would link users via the pre-existing Internet. Or, as information technology professionals describe it, the Web sits "on top of" the Internet.

Word of the CERN browser and the World Wide Web grew quickly within computing circles. In 1992 two of the staff at the National Center for Supercomputer Appliances at the University of Illinois at Urbana-Champaign showed the browser to computer science students. One of the students was a 22-year-old Midwesterner named Marc Andreessen, who was also a part-time employee of the center.

At that time, the Internet browser worked primarily only on Unix computers, one of the workhorses of computer operating systems, originally developed in 1969. Due to their expense, Unix machines were available for the most part only to large institutions.[10] (My how things have changed: today's operating system for Apple computers is based on a Unix platform; thus, the Apple system – one of the world's most popular computer brands – sits "on top of" the Unix platform.)

Andreessen recruited fellow NCSA employee Eric Bina to work on a user-friendlier browser that would work on other computer operating systems. The two worked all hours of the day and night and within months had a new browser they named Mosaic. Andreessen and Bina also devised new HTML tags that afforded more display and graphic options.

By early 1993, Mosaic for the Unix computing platform was available on NCSA's computers for downloading. Within weeks, tens of thousands of people had downloaded it. Andreessen and Bina feverishly started work on developing Mosaic for the PC and Mac/Apple, releasing those versions by spring of 1993.

10 http://bit.ly/OZWPPw

Mosaic became such a runaway success that the New York Times published a laudatory article about it on the front page of its business section in December of the same year – the same month, in fact, that Andreessen graduated from the University of Illinois. The Times article correctly predicted that Mosaic could launch "a new industry from scratch." The article mentioned neither Andreessen nor Bina, quoting only a handful of their professors. Further, Andreessen and Bina owned none of the fruits of their labor. Having been developed on university time, Mosaic was the property of the university rather than its creators.

After graduation, Andreessen moved to Mountain View, California, where he met Jim Clark, a 49-year-old founder of several successful technology companies. Andreessen combined his technical skills with Clark's money and connections to form Mosaic Communications Corporation in mid-1994. Andreessen recruited some friends from NCSA as employees with the goal to develop the next generation of browser. In October 1994, the Mosaic Netscape browser was posted for download on the Internet. It included yet more coding tags that permitted still greater design creativity.

Not so fast, said the University of Illinois, claiming that Andreessen had stolen its intellectual property. Over months of negotiations, the two parties reached a settlement: Mosaic Communications would change its name to Netscape and pay about $3 million for distribution rights to the university and for legal fees.

Next, Netscape went public with a stock offering in 1995, and by 1996, three of four users of the World Wide Web used a Netscape browser. In short order, of course, along came Microsoft with its Internet Explorer browser. A famous legal war ensued, lasting four years and involving the U.S. Department of Justice, 18 states and the District of Columbia. The plaintiffs' suit alleged that Microsoft was thwarting competition by forcing computer makers to include Internet Explorer as a part of the installation of Windows software.

Despite Netscape's successes and an ultimate judgment against Microsoft, the protracted struggle against Microsoft drained Netscape's resources, and in 1999 Netscape was sold to America Online for $10 billion in stock.[11] Today, Andreessen is an investor in and is on the board of directors for a number of technology companies including Facebook, Twitter and Digg. His net worth is estimated to be the same as that of two-time presidential candidate Mitt Romney. Not bad for a guy barely in his 40s.

Sorting through the jargon of today's Internet for practices

Let's put Internet history into the context of health care providers in private practice. Over the past decade, browser popularities and market shares have ebbed and flowed incessantly, as have computer operating systems. Additionally, the explosion of smart phones and computer tablets has transformed the computing landscape forever. All this

11 http://bit.ly/NuWvxJ

IT churning and burning spotlights a cold reality: It's becoming harder and harder for a medical practice to avoid having a presence on the World Wide Web.

The Internet allows innumerable modern conveniences, from scheduling an oil change for your car, to checking in on your family pet on Web cam at a doggie daycare center, to finding the nearest Ethiopian restaurant on a smart phone. Oddly, the medical profession – which hangs its hat on advances in health care technology – remains embarrassingly behind the information technology curve.

To see a doctor in the early 21st century, patients usually can only make an appointment through a phone call to the doctor's office during business hours – not counting the office's lunch "hour" between noon and 1:30 p.m. or even later. Once the patient has the appointment, she must then show up 20 minutes early fill out paperwork on a clipboard.

One reason that many professionals (not just physicians) have avoided a full plunge into the Internet is the baffling nature of the medium's jargon. Ironically, this is not at all unique to either information technology or to medicine. Like the medical profession, the IT world is punch-drunk on acronyms. This creates a chronic problem for medical practices just trying to manage the basics of their websites and get even a tenuous grasp on the perplexing array of acronyms such as SQL, PHP, and CSS.

Servers & clients & protocols, oh my

Every kind of device connected to the Internet – desktop computers, laptop computers, tablets and smart phones – is capable of receiving information over the Internet. By definition, any device receiving information is a client, and any device sending information to that client is a server. Conversely, the device receiving information could switch roles and become a server and send information to client devices elsewhere.

We saw earlier in this chapter that servers and clients have to follow rules in order to communicate. These rules include the transmission control protocol (TCP) and the Internet protocol (IP), courtesy of Kahn and Cerf, circa 1971. Each device connected to the Internet has its own IP address, which is how one computing machine can find another.

When an Internet user wants to look at a website, she enters a Web address into a browser window such as Internet Explorer or Mozilla Firefox or Google Chrome on her own computer monitor. Then, a Web page appears in the browser on her computer. Where does this page come from? Why, a Web server of course.

The server merely transmits its stored code for that particular website over the Internet to the computer of the person (client) requesting it.

Here is a sample of the code:

```
<!DOCTYPE html PUBLIC "-//W3C//DTD XHTML 1.0 Transitional//EN"
"http://www.w3.org/TR/xhtml1/DTD/xhtml1-transitional.dtd">

<html xmlns="http://www.w3.org/1999/xhtml" dir="ltr" lang="en-US">

<head profile="http://gmpg.org/xfn/11">

<title>IVF Atlanta Augusta Georgia Fertility</title>

<meta http-equiv="content-type" content="text/html" charset=UTF-8" />

<link rel='stylesheet' id='subpages-navigation-css'  href='http://ivfga.com/wp-content/plugins/subpage-navigation/subpage-navigation.css?ver=3.3.1' type='text/css' media='all' />
```

This is HTML code (hypertext markup language, discussed earlier), and this sample represents only about one-fiftieth of the code required to generate an elaborate website home page on a browser, but you get the idea. You can see the tags in the code, just like Caillau and Berners-Lee came up with back in 1990; for example, below are opening and closing title tags, which tells browsers to display the text in between:

```
<title>IVF Atlanta Augusta Georgia Fertility</title>
```

In addition to HTML code, most websites today use CSS code. This is short for "cascading style sheets," which looks like this:

```
h1 {

    color: white;

    text-shadow: 1px 1px 1px #222;

    font-weight: bold;

    line-height: 30px;

    font-size: 24px;

    margin-bottom: 10px;

}
```

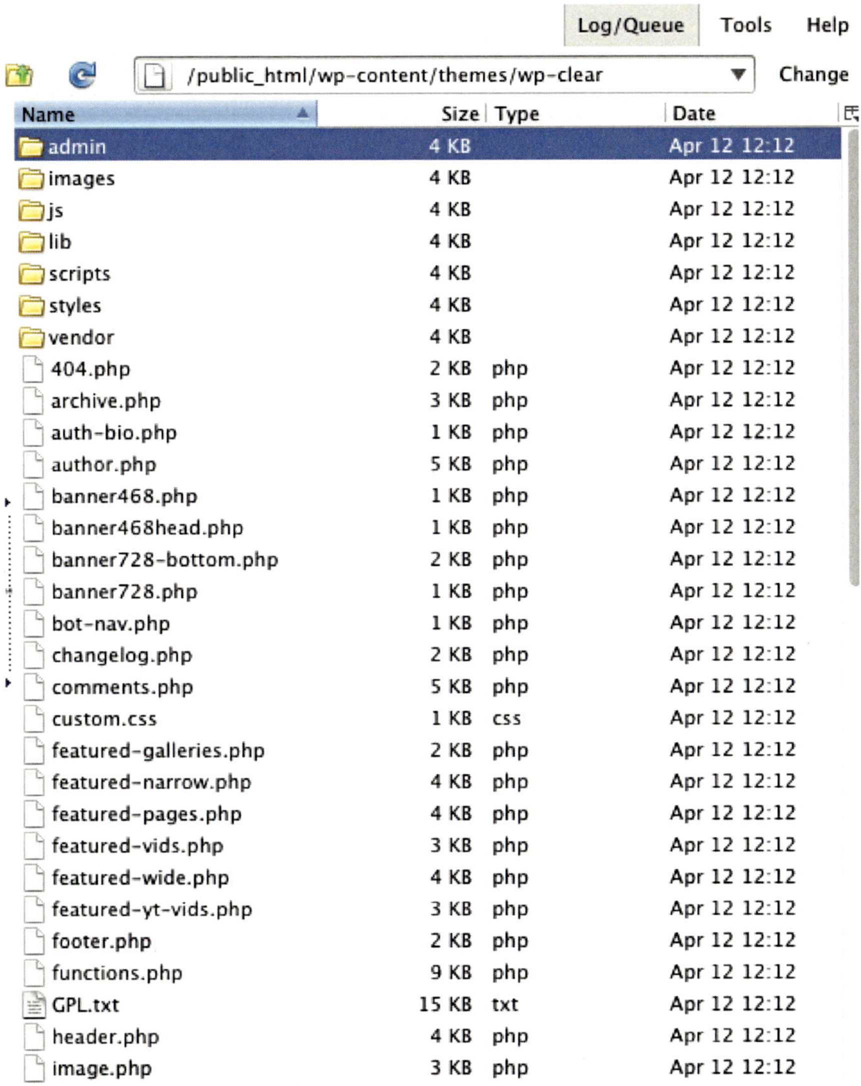

These are instructions to each client browser on how to render certain parts of the Web page. In this example, the code is telling a browser how to handle the color (make it white), style (bold), size, spacing and so on for all headline text tagged as an "H1" style – the largest of all headlines. Note also the similarity to opening and closing tags in HTML, except that CSS code uses opening and closing brackets like this: {code inside here}.

Each page on a website is typically stored as a separate file on a Web server, much like you might organize personal documents into separate files on your home computer. With certain software, you can look at a collection of documents making up a website, seeing something like the image above.

This is called a website directory (see graphic on previous page), and there is one exceptional trait about this collection of code documents that lives on a Web server:

Each document capable of generating a Web page is linked through code to other documents.

Why is this important? Because more and more, a single Web page today is actually an amalgam of multiple code documents. For example:

```
<a href="http://ivfga.com/patients/current-patients">

<img class="alignnone size-medium wp-image-1248" title="Current Patients
Button" src="http://ivfga.com/autothumb/image.php?src=/wp-content/up-
loads/2011/10/Current-Patients-Button-310x79.jpg&amp;aoe=1&amp;q=100&
amp;w=290&amp;h=74&amp;hash=e55272b49480d47d819102e4aa17cde1"
alt="Green button that says Current Patients, Click here for resource center" />

</a>
```

This is code in one document on a server telling a client browser to go to another file in the directory on that server titled "Current Patients Button" at the long Web address starting with "http://ivfga.com/autothumb..." and retrieve coding that produces a little green graphic doodad, resulting in the placement of that image (a button) on that web page.

Whew. Complicated enough? Wait, there's more! In fact, not all the documents making up a single Web page may reside on the same Web server. Often the document is a video file that resides on another server owned by a company called YouTube (or CBS News or the British Broadcasting Company or you name it). This is how video gets "embedded" in a Web page – the video lives on another website even though everything on that Web page doesn't come from that website. Indeed, one Web page may contain components sourced from dozens of other websites.

How stuff is found through Web addresses

With millions of computers on the Internet, how does a client computer find the one and only code document on the one and only server for a particular website? And how does one website find that single video it wants to embed amidst all the millions of other videos on YouTube? Through the domain name system (DNS).

Actually, the term DNS can be quite the source of aggravation to medical practice administrators and marketers and just about any other executives overseeing a business website. The topic usually raises its geeky little head just prior to a website launch or re-launch but also whenever there's a change in the site administration – when a new Web person or firm takes over a practice's website.

The domain name system is the phone book of the Internet. While we know websites by names such as WebMD.com and Google.com and NYTimes.com, true website addresses are located through servers assigned either 10- or 11-digit numbers such as 208.77.188.166. These number combinations are the bedrock of the Internet Protocol.

But what a pain it would be for Internet users to try to remember 10 or 11 digits to type in their browser address windows. Instead, we have the DNS, which allows us to use domain names such as Amazon.com. These kinds of Internet addresses, known as Uniform Resource Locators, or URL addresses, are worlds easier to remember than IP addresses. Now, whenever you type a URL into your browser window, a system of Web servers on the Internet looks up the IP address automatically and then knows where to send your request.

The DNS handles all this for you at nearly the speed of moving electrons. Consequently, any medical practice with a website needs a DNS account, much like a telephone account. This account is established with for-profit agencies accredited by the non-profit Internet Corporation for Assigned Names and Numbers (ICANN). Examples include GoDaddy.com, Register.com and MyHosting.com – formally known as DNS registrars.

So a medical practice can go to any of these agency websites and search for available names. If the DNS name that the practice wants - say, "GreatDoctors.com" - is available, the practice can reserve it for around $10 a year.

The name is reserved by filling out an online form asking for 1) a domain registrant (the practice in this case), 2) an administrative contact and 3) a technical contact. These contacts can be three different people or all the same person.

Probably the best approach is to register a practice shareholder or partner as the domain registrant and a Web specialist as the technical contact. That way, the account stays with the practice, while a more technically inclined delegate can handle the minutiae of administrating the account, including renewing the account when it comes due.

All of this is completely separate from hosting services. Registrars such as GoDaddy and MyHosting make their real money from offering website hosting on top of DNS registrations. Hosting a website (a server where the website code lives) can cost anywhere from $5 or $10 a month up to hundreds or even thousands of dollars monthly for extremely complex sites with heavy traffic.

Chapter 3

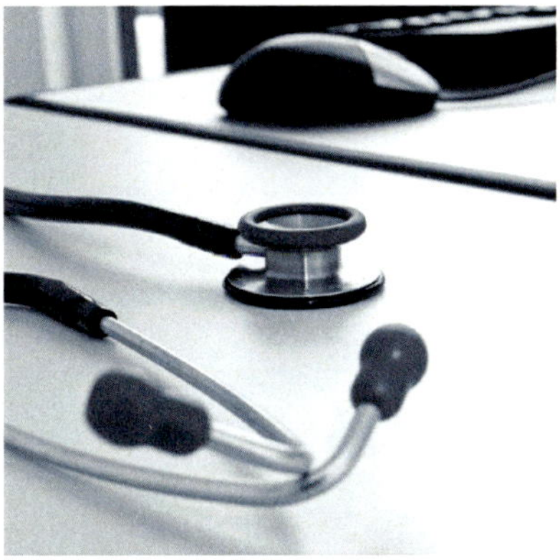

Doctors & patients

the last digital gap

In a May 2011 survey, the New York PR firm Makovsky + Company reported a notable finding: half of all Americans visit WebMD.com.[1] That this website is popular is not particularly surprising. What is surprising is just how popular. How many other websites can boast attracting half of a nation's population? WebMD is in very rare company in this distinction.

At the time, the survey also found that Facebook is the fourth most popular online resource for health care information, drawing one in nine Americans for that purpose. It has since risen to number two, according to the technology research company Alexa.[2] However, the key difference between WebMD and Facebook is significant: Physicians are the primary authors and sources on WebMD, while Facebook content is entirely what's called user-generated. In its survey, Makovsky + Company found that only 54 percent of survey respondents said they can rely on the accuracy of user-generated health information on social media sites such as Wikipedia, Facebook, Twitter, YouTube and blogs, compared with 68 percent saying they trust WebMD.

1 http://bit.ly/OECbs5

2 http://bit.ly/MWA27L

Further, the survey found that Web pages published by the U.S. government are the most trusted. Not surprisingly, websites sponsored or published by pharmaceutical companies are visited the least by Americans seeking health information (6 percent).

Notice anything missing here? Where is the survey question about health-information sites published by health care providers? Presumably, there are so few that it never occurred to the study sponsors to ask about them, which leads us to the true digital gap in medicine today.

The findings shouldn't surprise anyone but should give more credence to the idea that it's past time for health care providers to take a larger share of Internet voice. In the era of Facebook-fueled revolutions in the Arab world, it's hard to imagine an industry more behind the computer-and-Internet times than health care. In a 2009 survey of U.S. hospitals, the Harvard School of Public Health found that a mere 7.6 percent possessed even a basic EMR (electronic medical records) system.[3] A miniscule 1.5 percent had a comprehensive EMR. A year earlier, a similar survey of nearly 3,000 medical practices found only 13 percent of physicians in private practice had basic EMR systems and 4 percent had comprehensive systems.

Encouragingly, we seem to be on the verge of an upsurge in EMR adoption. Under the 2009 economic stimulus plan, the federal government will pay $44,000 per physician for EMR adoption. Mind you, to date much of this push for electronic records has been in the context of physician-to-physician usage: widespread EMR usage would theoretically enable the easy transfer of a patient's clinical records from one specialist to another.

The ubiquity of wired patients

All this bodes well for the health of patients. But what about the health of private medical practices? How do computer networks and digital data figure into the business equation of medicine?

For my money, a more interesting survey (assuming one has not been conducted) would be an assessment of the portion of medical practices with up-to-date websites, particularly Web 2.0 sites that allow patient-to-practice interaction and, probably more importantly, patient-to-patient interaction.

Is anyone not online these days? Consider:

> Four in five (80.6 percent) of American households have access to the Internet, according to the Pew Research Center.[4]

---

3 http://bit.ly/QP2FFq

4 http://bit.ly/OEDc3p

A nearly equal portion (85 percent) of Americans own cell phones, and six of 10 access the Internet wirelessly, according to Pew.

Pew reports that the fastest growing groups in Internet adoption are the elderly (in 2008-2009, Americans age 65-plus with home access to the Internet increased from 19 to 30 percent) and low-income households (with incomes between $20,000 and $40,000 annually), increasing from 42 to 53 percent in the same period).

So, in response to the question, is anyone not online these days, the clear answer is yes, too many doctors are not online, at least not with patients. It's time for catch-up.

Joining Web 2.0 conversations everywhere

Health care conversations and information seeking are everywhere out there on the 'Net, and for a physician to succeed in recruiting and retaining patients, s/he will have to be part of those conversations sooner than later. But too many doctors still cannot be easily found in a Google search.

In the free marketplace, consumers base choices on haves and have-nots. With time, more and more will gravitate to health care providers that have online accessibility. An established presence in the Web 2.0 world is no longer a luxury but a necessity for the practice of medicine, as essential as an exam room and a stethoscope. Successful competitors in the health care marketplace will have this; unsuccessful competitors will not.

Bottom line: Before long, doctors will have a simple choice – get wired or get retired. The forces of competition will guarantee it.

Part II

Marketing principles for medical practices

Chapter 4

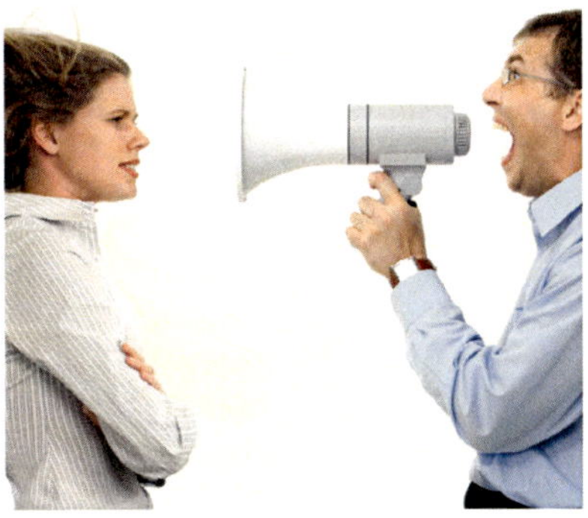

Meaning or noise?

Oh, what a difference

As useful as it is to learn about the Internet, it's more important to keep this fact in mind: it's only the medium.

Remember, the radio did not replace the newspaper; television did not kill off the radio; and the Internet hasn't done in TV (not yet anyway, although they perhaps are merging). Sorry, Marshall McLuhan, but there is a lot more message beyond any single medium, and in marketing, the message is everything. Here's why:

The first rule of marketing: Make the choice clear.

For medical practices, this means you want to create the impression in the minds of prospective patients: *There's medical practice XYZ* [your practice], *and then there's everyone else*.

Occupying a dominant place on the Internet by itself won't make that impression. Therein lies the fallacy of search engine marketing (covered in depth later). It's one thing to boost your website's search engine rankings so you'll fetch a lot of visitors to your website. It's quite another to "convert" a visitor, as we say in Web marketing – to turn a website visitor into a paying customer.

Customer conversion has everything to do with brand distinction. Just because I stroll by your luggage store in the shopping mall doesn't mean I'll march in and buy a suitcase. For that, you'll need a strong luggage brand. To have a strong brand, you need a good story. And a good story is about meaning, not noise.

The whisper heard 'round the world

On February 12, 2012, the burrito chain Chipotle made international news by airing its first national TV ad. It ran only once, on the Sunday-evening broadcast of the Grammy awards.

In just about any other circumstances, a company's first TV commercial would hardly merit a news story. This was different. The Chipotle ad generated headlines all over the country even before its television debut.

The fast-food industry spends more than $4 billion each year on advertising, most of it on TV. On television alone the average American child sees 15 food commercials every day, or approximately 5,500 commercials a year, according to Yale's Rudd Center on Food Policy and Obesity. [1]

Most TV commercials are 30 seconds long. The Chipotle TV spot was 2 minutes, 20 seconds – about five times longer.

Television's typical advertising fare features fast-moving, close-up shots of sizzling burgers or ribs or chicken fried in Lord-knows-what fatty substance. Instead, the Chipotle piece was an animation with a soundtrack, as country music legend Willie Nelson crooned his rendition of "The Scientist," a tune by the rock band Coldplay with no particularly overt meaning.

Remarkably, the advertiser's name didn't appear until 1 minute, 48 seconds into the production. When it finally did edge onto the screen, it was only a tiny logo incorporated almost imperceptibly into the animation. It disappeared 6 seconds later.

A simple message appeared at the conclusion: not "eat at Chipotle" or "our gourmet burritos are on sale this month" or "food with integrity," the company's slogan. Rather, the closing message was, "Cultivate a better world," a plug for Chipotle's foundation for supporting sustainable agriculture, family farming and culinary education. It wasn't even a commercial for Chipotle's food.

In addition to the single TV airing, Chipotle posted the animation to YouTube. In the first six months afterward, it averaged nearly a million viewings per month. Willie's crooning is also available on iTunes, where it has been downloaded so often that it has earned iTunes' highest popularity rating.

---

1 http://bit.ly/RNCNP8

David's burritos topples Goliath's burgers

Chipotle operates less than 1,300 stores worldwide – a fraction of the more than 5,600 Taco Bell locations and 23,000-plus Subway sandwich shops – but it's hardly struggling. The company's sales grew nearly 25 percent in 2011. Online magazine Slate has called Chipotle's 46-year-old founder, Steve Ells, the Steve Jobs of the restaurant industry. Time magazine lauded Ells for a building a company whose stock soared 800 percent in six years in part by persuading employees they are saving the world from obesity, tasteless food, chemicals and torture of animals.

Even so, how does a comparatively small fast-food company go up against a slew of competitors jamming 15 commercials into the average kid's day? Clearly, uniqueness is your only option.

Chipotle earns its distinctive place in the oh-so-crowded world of fast food by cultivating die-hard customer loyalty for its stated commitment to sustainable agriculture.

For example, it buys pork for its burritos from pigs that are raised outside on a vegetarian diet, and are not given antibiotics. On Halloween, Chipotle customers who dress up as a horrifying processed food are rewarded with a $2 burrito, with revenue going toward nutrition education.[2]

Chipotle's competitors, however, market the old-fashioned way. They shout. They fill the airways with blaring commercials showcasing the same old tacos, burgers and ribs.

Whereas most big fast-food sellers shout about their wares, Chipotle whispers. And people the world over listen. Why? Chipotle's messages have meaning to its audience.

Meaning is defined by personal values, needs, wants and/or beliefs and convictions. There's no shortage of humans with hard-fast values and convictions about how food should be grown and prepared.

You'd expect a fast-food chain to be the last to capitalize on those convictions. How utterly distinctive.

The end of shouting

Fifty years ago, when the U.S. population was barely half of today's census, a marketer could reach about 75 percent of the population just by advertising for a week on a half-hour nightly news program on one of the three national TV networks.

That was then. This is now, with 500-plus channels now on cable TV and somewhere around 300 million websites. Chipotle has made its products such a clear choice that

2 http://bit.ly/NJLia2

airing just one TV commercial generates hundreds of thousands of YouTube visits each week.

Chipotle's messages have meaning, which is defined by personal values, needs, wants and/or beliefs and convictions. There's no shortage of humans with hard-fast values and convictions about how food should be grown and prepared.

There are two lessons here for medical practices. First, in most cases, advertising a practice the traditional way in newspapers or on TV or billboards just won't get you a lot. The marketplace is already too noisy out there for you to be heard above the din of 15 fast-food commercials daily. If you advertise, you're competing not so much against other health care providers but more against all the other advertisers in the cacophonous public space.

Secondly, be unique. Then talk about it, on your website, in your brochures, on your on-hold telephone messages, and at every possible touch point with patients.

A caveat: even if a medical practice avoids the costly option of traditional advertising, branding still takes resources. New patients don't come free or even cheap. You're going to have to pay for them.

But what's the alternative? Going head to head on TV against McDonald's and Wendy's? Don't even try. You'll strain your voice trying to shout that loud.

Chapter 5

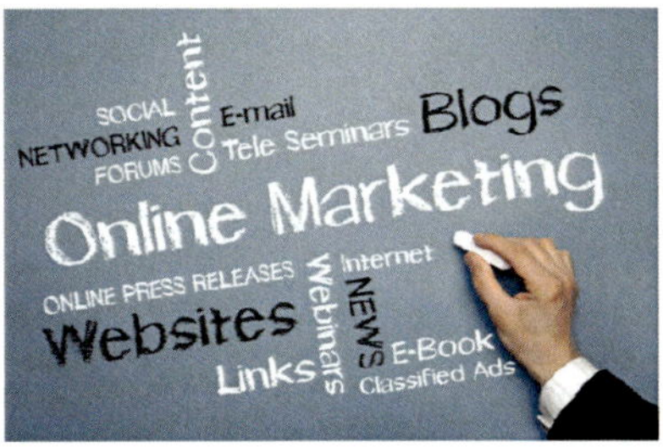

Marketing, branding, advertising, PR...

what's the diff?

In my professional experience over the last 15 years, I've found considerable confusion in the medical profession over marketing nomenclature. One person's definition of public relations or branding may vary wildly from another's.

Here, in my opinion, are the most important and relevant marketing terms and their definitions:

Marketing communications include both the message and the media of advertising. For the media, you can choose among advertising (TV, newspapers, magazines, radio, etc.), the Internet and public relations, among other options

The **target audience** in marketing communications is generally your customers, although it often also includes non-customers who can influence your customers. For medical specialists, primary care physicians are an example of the latter.

Advertising requires you to pay for space for your message to appear to target audiences in print and Internet media, or for time to broadcast it on radio and TV.

Public relations (PR) is the discipline of inspiring your target audiences and/or audience influencers to talk favorably about your products or services. Public relations used to center on the pursuit of favorable coverage in the mainstream news media. Increasingly, PR focuses on social media and self-publishing on the Internet.

Branding is communicating the distinctions of your products or services.

In discussing these concepts with people who aren't professional marketers, I've generally found that most folks fall into one of two philosophical camps.

In the first camp are those who feel overwhelmed and mystified by marketing, a voodoo art totally beyond their comprehension or rational understanding.

In camp two are the cake decorators. For them, marketing is a matter of making whatever you do look really pretty and pushing it out there in front of buyers. Put enough icing on it and make sure it comes in a nice box with a bow on top, and customers will pay for it. After all, what you do is so great and irresistible, who wouldn't want to buy it, right?

Folks in camp two aren't entirely wrong. There's a reason Godiva chocolates come in a box, while Hershey's bars come wrapped in faux foil. You pay more for Godiva, so it looks like it's more expensive.

Yes, but ... there really is more to it than that. What Godiva promises – like all successful brands – is a special experience. The box certainly is part of it, but not all. Notice that Godiva has a slogan proudly proclaiming its Belgian tradition dating back to 1836. In the United States, if it's gourmet food imported from Europe, the common assumption is that it must be better, especially if it costs more.

More precisely, Godiva treats its product as a scarce and valuable indulgence. Look on its website for this very message, from Godiva's "chocolatier," Monsieur Thierry Muret: (quel savant!):

> *According to Muret, fine chocolates are more expensive because they cost more to make. Their intensity of aroma, texture and flavor, however, means that people can easily satisfy their chocolate cravings with only one or two pieces, making fine chocolates one of life's affordable luxuries.*

Just like diamond rings and Ben & Jerry's ice cream, Godiva chocolates are sold in small portions. These products all must be valuable, or else you could buy them in big bags like you buy unshelled peanuts at the county fairgrounds or "family value size" paper napkins at Costco.

Godiva is exemplary in following the first rule of marketing. They stand out from the pack. Google the word "chocolate" and you'll get nearly a billion results. Godiva's right there on the first page, along with Ghiradelli, another gourmet chocolate that stands out from the pack.

Yes, Hershey is also on page one of Google results, but for a different reason. Godiva and Ghiradelli both have stories, both geographical in this instance: Godiva's story is European gourmet, and Ghiradelli's story is San Francisco "premium."

The stories are nearly identical. All it takes is one key distinction to make a compellingly different story. Do you want Euro gourmet or San Fran gourmet? Chocolate lovers know and remember the difference well enough to buy lots of both.

Sentenced to 20 years of boredom

In contrast, Hershey doesn't have a real story. It has ubiquity. It's everywhere. I dare you to find a convenience store or gas station in the United States that does not sell fist-size Hershey's bars for a couple of bucks or less, packing enough sucrose to knock a 300-pound NFL linebacker into a stupor.

All three chocolate makers have successful marketing. But only two really have stories. Godiva and Ghiradelli have value precisely because you cannot find them in every juke joint in America. In place of a story, Hershey has noise.

These examples emphasize a fundamental truth:

In marketing you have only three choices –

1. Boredom
2. Shouting
3. Seduction

Most businesses are forced into boredom-based marketing. They just don't have the product distinction or the marketing budget to build a mass of die-hard, loyal customers quickly.

This includes lots of locally or regionally based gourmet chocolate makers. They have a widely recognized brand name in certain cities or states or regions to draw just enough customers for modest success, but not enough to have what we'd call a global brand name. They spend 10, 20 or 50 years barely making a blip on the national scene.

It's not their fault that they're not very famous. It's hard to find fame. But to be famous, you have to be famous for something. And most local brands haven't found their fame hook yet – that one story that spreads like wildfire on its own because customers can't help but retell the story to others and thereby create new customers.

Some luckier businesses are able to select the second choice, shouting. This group often includes car dealers and warehouse furniture marts. These retailers churn so much merchandise volume and gross so many dollars of sales that they've got the bucks to blast their way onto the airwaves of radio and TV and onto display ads on popular websites.

Unless you live in a cave, you can't shut these shouters out of your life. Their advertisements saturate the mass media, and you wish you could just forget their names and their jingles, but you can't.

Why don't they just shut up? I'll tell you why. Shouting works. You can't forget oft-shouted names even when you want to. In the marketing business this is called top of mind. Not being able to get something out of your mind can be a huge asset to the seller who put it there.

It's my duty to report with regret that more and more doctors are becoming shouters. For reasons to be shared later, I think doctor shouting is neither becoming to the profession nor cost effective. An infinitely better alternative is seduction, the third choice of marketing.

Seduction is the purview of masters such as Fred Smith (founder of FedEx), Calvin Klein (fashion designer) and Steve Jobs (co-founder of Apple Electronics). Each was able to devise a great brand built on making the clearest of all choices to their customers. The seduction is so strong that all it takes is a whisper to generate customers sleeping out on the sidewalks in front of Apple stores the world over on the night before the newest iWhatever goes on sale.

The choices put forth by these masters was so clear that each was able to boil their distinctions down to a word or two: "overnight" for Smith, "rustic elegance" for Klein, and "hip simplicity" for Jobs. Each inspired unique feelings in their customers that no competitor inspired.

Nobody feels quite the same way about the United States Postal Service Express Mail as they feel about FedEx. And Apple iPads, iPhones, iTunes ... well, big Steve transcended all previous brand legends, looming ever larger in death than he did even in life.

Alright, so now you're asking, *What in heaven's name do any of these ideas have to do with medical practices? I'm in the business of prostate surgeries or spinal fusions, not peddling tablet computers.*

Good point. Many of the broad concepts of branding can apply to medical practices. There's a lot to learn and apply from the world of mainstream consumer products and services.

Chapter 6

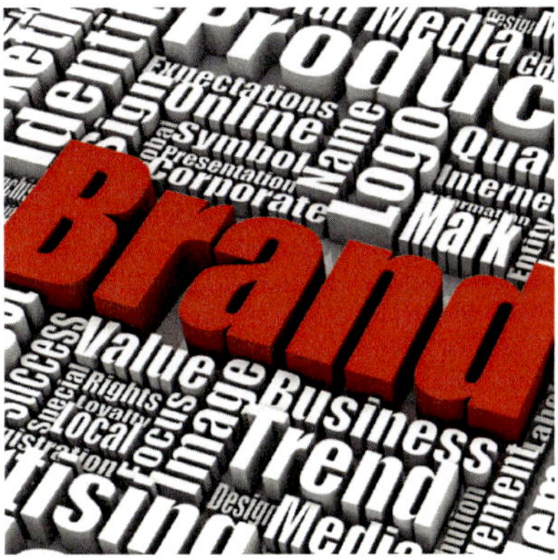

Brand building for medical practices

You hear the word "brand" thrown around so much these days that it's easy to wonder if it has meaning any more. You also may wonder what it has to do with growing a medical practice.

Branding is a matter of new curiosity to medical practices, even though brands seep into our lives from birth. Typically, by the time a child enters third or fourth grade, s/he knows what makes a Corvette different from a Dodge Caravan, and where in the grocery store to find Ben & Jerry's products.

But can a medical practice have a brand? If so, what is a doctor or a practice administrator supposed to do with it?

Excellent questions. To find answers, it helps to have a definition: A brand is simply a claim of distinction, and the reason any organization needs one is for business health. Every organization exists to provide products or services or both, even if the organization is a professional-services group or a non-profit.

Those products and services must be relevant to the organization's customers or constituents – they must be meaningful to both heads and hearts. You can't merely say or even prove your product or service is better than most. You have to make consumers believe and feel it.

Size doesn't matter. Distinctions do.

The most successful organizations usually have a strong brand that clearly differentiates them from all competitors.

Brands are not a function of organizational size or market dominance. Chevrolet is one of the world's largest automakers, yet Volvo and Rolls Royce are stronger brands (for different reasons), more easily associated with clear distinctions.

Similarly, Apple computers and electronics, Ikea furnishings and Swiss Army Knives don't outsell all competitors but nonetheless cultivate legions of till-death-do-us-part customers. A seller can't buy such loyalty; he or she must earn it by staking out clear distinctions.

The first impression is the most important, and it must make the choice clear. Specifically, what can be said about a private medical practice that is not true about others? In the free market, every health care provider faces three essential questions:

1. *Are you really different?*

2. *How?*

3. *Who else knows it?*

Often – perhaps even most of the time – the smallest of distinctions will build a strong brand. Volvo originally made the branding claim of safety because in the 1980s they were the first European automaker to include seat belts as standard equipment. But does Volvo actually make the safest car?

In late 2011, Subaru was the first carmaker able to say that all its models earned the title of Top Safety Pick by the Insurance Institute of Highway Safety.[1] Barely half of Volvo's nine models got the same designation for 2012.

Yet after three decades of branding itself as the safe car, Volvo still owns that category in the minds of car buyers.

There are generally two kinds of brands:

An **inherent brand** is built inextricably into the product or service for sale. Of the products we've covered so far in our discussion of branding, Apple computers and Rolls Royce automobiles are two examples of this kind of brand, for different reasons. Unlike PCs, Apple computers have proprietary software that no other manufacturer can sell.

1 http://bit.ly/LNCIsg

Rolls Royce's branding is built into its price tag; at around $250,000 per car, the carmaker can afford to offer the most luxurious of products.

A **derived brand** comes from a deliberate effort to distinguish a product or service outside its own traits. An excellent example is Frontier Airlines, a Colorado-based regional carrier that has survived various ups and downs of the airline industry in part by putting cute pictures of animals on its airplane tails – bobcats, bears, and dolphins, among others. Frontier has quite a few loyal customers who can hardly wait for the next flight, just to see what animal adorns their jet. Otherwise, Frontier isn't much different from other airlines.

In the health care sector, medical practices tend to focus on inherent brands, usually some specialty-related distinction in each marketplace. An example might be advanced radiation equipment that has been licensed exclusively to one oncology practice in one city for a limited period of, say, three years.

Such a clear distinction could make for strong branding for as long as the exclusivity lasts – or until the practice can find another technological distinction when the three years are up. However, there are other paths to branding success, each worthy of examination.

Branding path one: Durable simplicity

The good news is that, in order to be successful, a medical practice rarely needs an entirely unique distinction. It isn't necessarily a requirement for effective branding in any industry, perhaps less so for practices. Sometimes you just have to be first to make the claim, just as Volvo has done.

Fortunately, almost all practices have to compete only in their metropolitan area, not nationally or even regionally or statewide. It's not so hard to be unique amid a handful or, at most, a few dozen competitors in one city.

In our experience in specialty medicine, examples have included:

> An orthopedics practice with the largest staff of physical and occupational therapists within 100 miles.
>
> A neurosurgery group that offers the widest range of minimally invasive surgeries for degenerative disc disease of the lumbar spine, thus eliminating overnight hospital stays.
>
> A fertility practice with a special arrangement with far-flung OB/GYNs willing to monitor induced ovulation procedures so that female patients wouldn't have to travel far for daily sonograms.

At the same time, keep in mind the risks of building a brand around a single physician or surgical procedure. What if the physician leaves the group? What if your competitors learn the same procedure? What if a splashy research study later triggers widespread doubt as to the safety of the procedure?

The key is broad and durable simplicity. Ideally, you want to say something about your practice that's succinct, compelling and hard to imitate. Don't try to build a brand around multiple strengths. Yes, Starbucks sells sandwiches and salads, but its brand is associated with special coffee.

Pick the strongest, most lasting distinction to patients (not to other doctors) and fly that flag high. Repeat the message on your office door, your business cards, your website, even on your lab coats. Wear it with pride. Above all, make in stick in the minds of health care consumers.

Branding path two: Solidly in first place

Often a medical practice was the first to achieve a notable medical accomplishment in its area, or is the oldest in its specialty, or has the most of something that it will probably never lose.

For example, my consulting firm has a client practice in fertility medicine that enabled one of the first births through *in vitro* fertilization on the West Coast, and also helped deliver the second baby born in the United States from a previously frozen embryo. Note that the practice was not first in either category nationally. It doesn't have to be.

The nature of health care is that it's a locally provided service. Ninety-nine percent of patients want appointments with doctors in their hometowns. This is particularly true in the IVF specialty, which requires women to undergo a series of treatments, monitoring and procedures, sometimes even on a daily basis.

This same client practice of ours is also responsible for more than 5,000 IVF births in its 30-year history. Prospective patients in the same state have to travel a long ways to find another practice with that kind of track record.

Branding path three: Actionable promises

Be careful to avoid the most common trap for medical practices: You can't be unique by merely saying you excel in patient care. Every patient expects that. Just about every medical practice says it.

The strongest brands are built on distinguished and unarguable customer experiences. Sometimes all it takes is having a silly picture of a wild critter on the tail of the airplane to make a passenger feel special about being inside the plane. Every driver of a Mercedes-Benz looks straight through the windshield and down the hood at the metal, tripod-inside-a-circle logo mounted in the most prominently visible location on the automobile. The experience constantly reinforces the driver's pride in piloting one of the world's most prestigious brands.

If you're offering the special experience of exceptional patient care, by far the better action is to prove it. Words without action don't mean much. Deeds count. If you don't believe it, go read reviews of doctors on rate-your-doctor websites such as Yelp.com and Vitals.com. The worst complaints are often from former patients who got sick of spending 45 minutes in the waiting rooms of medical practices that promised "excellence in care" or something like it.

Examples of actionable uniqueness include:

- Giving patients online access to some of their medical records.
- Guaranteeing on your website that no patient has to wait 15 minutes before seeing a provider.
- Offering free public seminars on conditions your practice treats.

Yep, any and all of these distinctions take time, money and commitment. But only a minority of practices offers such provable experiences. In most cities, a practice would be unique in its specialty by offering any two, sometimes just one.

Branding path four: Get professional help

The lament of marketing professionals everywhere is that few people without the professional training or experience claim to be qualified to practice medicine, but everyone thinks s/he's a marketer. I thought that, too, before I actually became one.

Once I became a full-time marketer, I ran headfirst into another stonewall: doing your own marketing is like doing your own surgery. When you're that close to the action, there is too much you just can't see as well as an outsider can.

It's a fact that the higher you rise in any organization and the more responsibility you take on, the farther you are from the customer's point of view. You suffer from too many executive biases and blinders. You have the curse of knowledge – you know too much about how it should be for you, the seller, rather than for them, the buyers.

Take it from a seasoned pro: branding strategy is the hardest and most often screwed-up part of marketing. The more years I acquire of branding experience as a consultant, the more respectful I am of its difficulty.

The most powerful brands are usually drawn from a combination of three forces: buyer needs and wants, a seller's offerings, and the seller's inherent tradition and culture. Everything that made Apple computers and Volvo automobiles what they are as brands came directly from the personality traits of Steve Jobs and the centuries-old culture of Sweden, where icy roads and a strong sense of social responsibility gave birth to the car's brand built on safety.

There are core cultural differences – motivating convictions and values – between the organizations founded by Steve Jobs and Bill Gates (of Microsoft), just as there are sharp cultural distinctions between Gothenburg, Sweden (location of Volvo's worldwide headquarters), and Detroit, Michigan. The products from each seller reflect those distinctions. The intuitive skills and wisdom required to discern the distinctions – and then distill them into messages that hit the target audience where they live – are akin to those required to write a classic novel or carve a sculpture that winds up at the Louvre a century later.

Legend has it that it used to take Pablo Picasso less than 10 minutes to do one of his famous pen-and-ink renderings of a bull fight that now fetch hundreds of thousands of dollars. Picasso's purported response: "It took me 50 years to do a drawing in 10 minutes."

My honest advice is, don't try to do your own surgery. Dialing in your brand correctly will boost your business and revenues for years to come. Don't try this at home on your own. Buy the right expertise just once and you'll never regret it.

Chapter 7

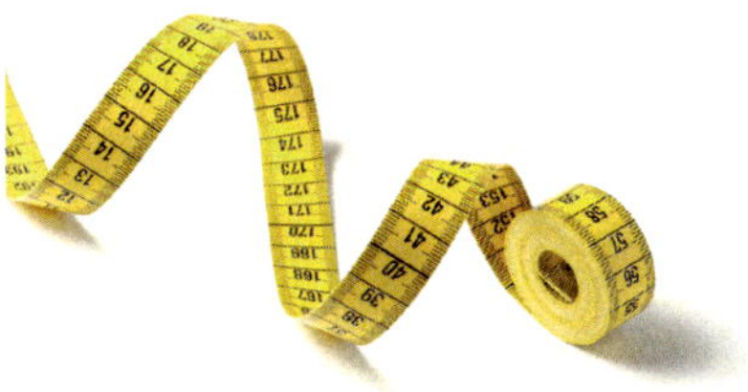

Measuring marketing:

the good, the bad & the unachievable

To some people on the outside, marketing doesn't look all that hard. Maybe you're one of those people. If, after reading the previous chapters, you're still in the cake-decorating camp, consider this: Marketing is principally the art and sometimes science of changing human behavior. What's so easy about that?

The goal in marketing is to affect consumer choices. How do you know when it succeeds? If sales/revenues/new-patient volumes go up, how do you know why? How do you measure cause and effect in human behavior? If a new patient comes to a medical practice, can you say with certainty that it was 40 percent because she liked that practice's website and 60 percent because her sister is already a patient?

Non-marketers frequently want to believe in simple answers to these questions. In medicine, traditionally there has been one simple answer – a patient sees a certain specialist because her primary care physician told her to. If you manage a practice and want to live solely off physician referrals, I've already warned you in the foreword to stop reading, and shame on you for coming this far.

For everyone else, rarely are there simple answers to the above questions, even when a new patient says unequivocally, "I picked your practice because of its website!" Don't automatically believe it. Why exactly do humans do what they do? When did you decide blue was your favorite color and why? At what precise point did your spouse decide you were the one? Do you recall the hour, date and place you decided Meryl Streep or Dustin Hoffman is the greatest actor of all time? It's hard to get reliable answers from the humans themselves. Do they always want to admit to their motivations? How often do they really know?

Nonetheless, the 21st century has brought some good news: One of the Internet's marvelous benefits is that it allows much more measurement of human behavior. We'll look at this in detail in later chapters. For now, suffice to say that we can attach many more numbers to human behavior in terms of website visits, responses to Internet ads, and so on, than we've ever been able to do before.

At the same time, not everything happens on the Internet or is measurable there. You may get a new patient not just because her sister is already a patient, but also because the new patient also visited a rate-your-doctor website or your practice's Facebook page or spoke to a neighbor and liked what she saw or heard in any of those places.

Fact is, these are all contributors to this thing called marketing noise, and noise does indeed contribute to marketing success. Any medical practice marketing directly to consumers needs a certain level of noise. Where it gets tough is knowing where to buy that noise.

No question in business has created more anxieties and hand wringing than this one: What's the wisest use of my marketing dollar? Herewith are three methodologies for ascertaining at least an educated guess.

Three key metrics in medical marketing

1. Outbound communications: The oldest and most common marketing metric centers on how much noise you're making. The traditional metric was CPM, or cost per thousand – how many dollars does it cost to send your marketing message to 1,000 recipients?

Pros: This measure fits well into old-fashioned advertising. Television networks and newspaper publishers spend zillions on independent audits to prove how many people are watching each TV show (courtesy of The Nielsen Company) or reading each copy of the daily newspaper (the Audit Bureau of Circulations).

Cons: Outbound measurements tell you only how much noise you made, not how many people responded or even why they responded. For all you know, every one of those TV watchers Tivo-ed right through your commercial.

2. Inbound response: We like this kind of metric because it can reveal how many people reacted to your pitch. If you pay for a 60-second commercial on skin rejuvenation at the low, low price of $99.95 and have viewers call a special toll-free number, you're able to count every caller.

Pros: With the help of special telephone tracking numbers and website addresses, it's gotten very easy to run these kinds of marketing campaigns. Website analytics also open up a whole new universe of insights into consumer behavior. (See the next section for more.)

Cons: Medicine rarely fits the direct-response marketing model. Patients seek treatment mainly when they need it, not when a health care provider offers it. Medical practices aren't selling beer and potato chips, the products in the category of so-called impulse buying.

3. Anecdotal feedback: Sometimes all it takes is hearing from a few very satisfied customers (patients) to know when you've struck gold. There's nothing like personal feedback to ring your bell.

An insightful experience, repeated many times: My firm spends more than 100 hours annually gathering data to show return on our marketing efforts to each client medical practice. "That's nice," the doctors often respond. "But how do I know these patients wouldn't have found us anyway?"

The fact is, some of them no doubt would have. But not all. And that's where the arguing starts – how many exactly can the marketing department claim credit for? Then, by gosh and by golly, as soon as one or two physicians in the same practice hear from, say, two or three new patients within a week or two that their brilliant new website was the reason those patients booked appointments, then that website was worth every penny!

Pros: See immediately above.

Cons: This is the least scientific way to measure return. But hey, as long as you feel like you made the right choice, enjoy it while it lasts, especially if the other two metrics support it.

Eat your vegetables

If all this feels less than totally satisfying, perhaps it's a consolation to know that titans of industry have wrestled with the questions of marketing metrics for decades. To date, no one seems to have found an encompassing answer to satisfy all questions.

A famous saying has been attributed to various celebrity entrepreneurs: I know I'm wasting half of my marketing dollar; I just don't know which half.

Most have come to a peaceful acceptance of some level of mystery. This concept shouldn't be foreign to physicians. How much of medicine and advice to patients is educated guessing? Plenty, despite a massive body of medical knowledge and decades of supporting clinical data.

Yes, we can predict fairly closely, for example, how many colorectal cancer patients will still be alive five years after treatment with 5-Fluorouracil, a first-choice chemotherapy treatment that has been through a multitude of clinical trials with proven success. But exactly which patients will still be alive? And what do we tell patients about avoiding colorectal cancer to start with?

On that latter question, the first response of oncologists is that genetics are everything in determining cancer destiny, and so take care to pick your parents carefully. Very funny.

Their next tip is to focus on a healthy lifestyle of vigorous exercise and a diverse diet that includes fruits and vegetables. Sure thing. Does that mean three servings a day, like we were told as kids? Or should it be the more current recommendation of five servings a day? Should we limit red-meat consumption to once a week, once a month, or not at all? Are three gym visits a week enough to stop cancer, or is five better? Come on, which is it?

Face it: nobody knows. Nobody probably ever will, not with absolute conclusiveness. And so it is with the individual components of marketing noise. The sensible approach is to continue to generate noise, measure output and input the best you can, and then make adjustments based on the best educated guesses possible. Meanwhile, make peace with knowing you'll never quite attain the elusive goal of certainty.

Chapter 8

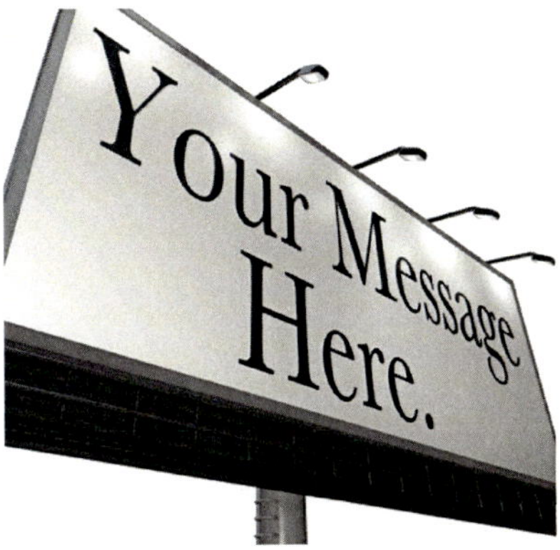

Beware the sirens of advertising

By now it should be abundantly clear that successful branding does not depend on noise. Rather, it's largely the opposite. The stronger your brand, the less noise you will probably need in order to tell your target audience about it.

The most visible and oldest form of mass marketing noise is traditional advertising. A lot of doctors advertise. It seems that more are advertising than ever before, raising this question: In medicine, when is traditional advertising a good idea for a specialty medical practice? Good question. Easy answer: Just about never.

Reason one is credibility. According to a Harris poll, only one in five American adults say they trust that advertising is honest in its claims all or most of the time (19 percent). About two-thirds of Americans (65 percent) say they trust that advertising is sometimes honest in its claims, while about one in ten (13 percent) say that they never trust that advertising is honest in its claims.

Do the math. If you advertise, you've got between a one-in-five and a two-in-three chance you'll be believed. Are those good enough odds for a medical practice? Possibly, although the odds are less attractive when you factor in the unique role that trust plays in health care.

When it comes to their bodies, humans can be far more skeptical about commercial messages. For serious health matters, they want a highly competent doctor, which is an entirely different purchase decision than buying chocolate or a burrito. Remember, picking a doctor is what professional marketers call a considered purchase, requiring careful consideration.

Reason two is measurability. As you can infer from the previous chapter, noise is only easy to gauge in an outbound context. It can be quite difficult to measure in terms of inbound response, though certainly possible if you use special telephone numbers and website addresses for tracking response.

Even so, beware the advertising sirens. They're youthful, they're gorgeous, and they sing alluringly. For medical practices, they're also seducers who can lure innocents to financial waste.

The appeal of mass media is strong. It's human nature to revel at the sight of your own name in lights. For this reason, physicians can drift almost helplessly toward the purchase of public exposure on billboards, television, and in magazines and newspapers.

This temptation becomes even stronger when a competitor suddenly appears in any of these media. By nature, physicians are hyper-competitive. They have to be in order to pass all the pressure-intensive auditions of a medical education and professional training.

Thus, discovering a cross-town rival's ad on TV or in the local newspaper trips a doctor's competitive alarm. "I'd better respond," is his or her gut instinct. "I need an ad, too. A bigger, better ad!"

Before you get out the checkbook, consider:

Mathematics – How many motorists passing a billboard every day are contemplating fertility treatments or a hip replacement? How many TV viewers are suffering from kidney stones or prostate cancer?

A tiny percentage, that's how many. One in 20 would be a surprisingly high number. At this rate, you the advertiser are throwing away 95 cents of every dollar you spent on your ad to talk to otherwise healthy people reaching for the radio dial or the mute button.

Yes, in most cases so many people see a billboard or TV commercial that you will indeed reach some people who fit the very narrow demographics of your next patient – if you spend enough money to own the best advertising time and space. But there are better, cheaper ways to find new patients.

Intrusion – Consumers run away from advertising. They regard it as an annoying interruption. Why do you think people pay for Tivo machines and high-speed Internet connections? For them, advertising equals unwanted propaganda.

When you factor in advertising's credibility problem, the math gets even worse. A survey by Adweek Media/Harris Poll found that only one in five Americans believe advertising is honest in its claims most or all of the time.[1] So even if you're okay with a 5-percent efficiency in reaching your target audience (see above), of that 5 percent, 4 percentage points of that audience still may not believe your paid message. So now we're down to 1 percent return on investment. Ugh.

The Internet – While the odds of your next patient driving by a billboard with your name on it is modest at best, the odds of your next patient (or a loved one acting on his or behalf) going on the Internet are virtually certain.

You simply cannot under-estimate the power of pull communications (answering a need or question) versus intrusion advertising. People who need a medical specialist WILL go online at one point or another – usually to look for health information first and then a health provider second.

Pull, not push, new patients

Of course, there are always exceptions to any rule of thumb. In certain circumstances some forms of noise can be cost effective. For a few medical specialties, community sponsorships are a good idea, when the sponsorships reach highly targeted audiences. Examples include support for relevant community events (e.g., kids events for pediatric sponsors), public radio and TV (for specialties focused on middle-age and older patients), and sports teams (appropriate for orthopedists).

But reasonable returns on investments in medical mass-media advertising are rare in most situations. In fact, the difficulty of measuring returns is one of the drawbacks to traditional advertising. As you would expect to read in a book about the power of the Internet, the evidence is overpowering that far better returns are possible with online communications and marketing, the physician's best friend for reaching the most patients and prospective patients for the lowest cost.

There are two reasons for these: publishing cost and audience media habits.

Before the Internet, the traditional broadcast and print media (radio, television, newspapers, magazines) largely controlled communications access to the masses because they controlled distribution channels. Back in the 20th century, it took a fortune to build a TV or radio station, with all that expensive studio and broadcasting equipment, including massive towers that would reach into the sky far enough to send out a strong signal.

Similarly, to be successful in the newspaper business, you had to own a titanic printing press and a fleet of trucks and hire an army of drivers and newspaper boys and girls on bicycles to deliver the finished product to every customer's door. Magazine publishers

1 http://bit.ly/M8Da5N

usually leased printing presses to print each edition, typically at costs of hundreds of thousands of dollars for a national readership. Distribution via mail to subscribers' homes and shipping to newsstands tacked on hundreds of thousands more to the cost of doing business.

Then came cable TV and the high-speed Internet into American homes, and poof, distribution costs fall to a tiny fraction. Suddenly, the price of being a publisher or broadcaster plummets to nearly nothing. You can even shoot video on your $100 cell phone, upload it to YouTube and be in the broadcasting business in minutes.

Technology has turned the doctor, dentist, baker and candlestick maker into publishers and broadcasters the world over. Glory, glory, hallelujah. Fueled by Internet search engines, websites can now put almost anyone in touch with almost anyone else at fractional costs, even a sustenance farmer in Bhutan, as we saw in Part I.

As to audience habits, consider: As of 2006, seven in 10 Americans with household incomes of at least $75,000 annually had high speed Internet access at home, according to the Pew Research Center.[2] And the percentage of those who look for health information online? About nine in 10. Those portions have no doubt increased in the five years since.

Do the math again. You'll see that about four out of five of the best patients – the ones with the education and the means to seek medical treatment and have the best outcomes – are online.

The next time you hear the sirens' song, proceed cautiously. As lovely as the sound may be, their tune may only siphon time, energy and dollars far better spent elsewhere – namely, on meaningful information and communications with patients. We explore the more effective alternatives in the next section, on the many and wondrous facets of the Internet and social media.

2 http://bit.ly/NuXaz7

Part III

Growing a practice through online conversations

Chapter 9

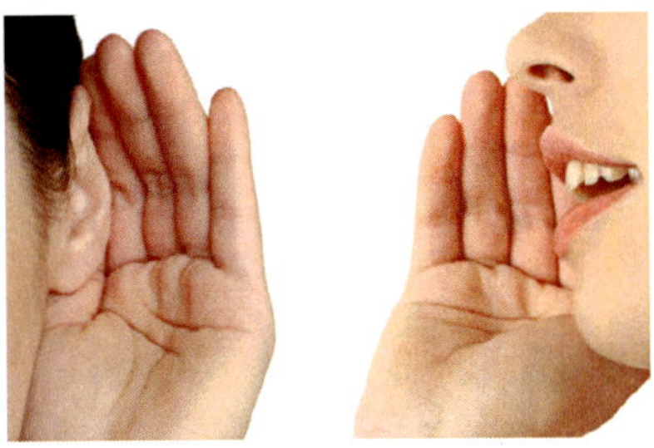

Medical marketing as conversation

Health care crowdsourcing

A magnificent convenience of living on an Internet-connected planet is having access to global inventories. If you want it, you can find it on the 'Net in bountiful quantities, and chances are you'll pay a fraction of the price you would have paid a decade ago – regardless of what it is.

Wired magazine documented the phenomenal rise of global accessibility in June 2006, when it published an article on the then-new trend called crowdsourcing.[1] In the article, writer Jeff Howe noted that in pre-Internet days, a successful professional photographer could easily command hundreds or thousands of dollars each time someone wanted to publish one of that photographer's images.

Then came search engines and the two-way communications benefits of Web 2.0, allowing Internet users to browse millions of high-quality photographs for sale on stock-photo websites for a few bucks each. Howe's article cited the case of a project director at the National Health Museum willing to pay as much as $600 each for professionally shot

1 http://bit.ly/NJLTbJ

photos of people sneezing and coughing – until the project director discovered an online stock house, where she downloaded 56 such photos for about $1 each.

"Technological advances in everything from product design software to digital video cameras are breaking down the cost barriers that once separated amateurs from professionals," Howe wrote.

So it is for just about any product or service. Any customer of almost anything can often put out what amounts to a request for a bid and typically have hundreds or thousands of responses, often in minutes or less. This is crowdsourcing.

Crowdsourcing today is such an accepted habit that some call it an industry – notably the websites crowdsourcing.org and crowdsourcing.com. The latter website asserts glibly, "the crowd is driving the future of business."

Industry or not, one could make a pretty good argument that crowdsourcing is driving present health care, and that more medical practices should take advantage of it.

Playing a doctor on the Internet

The notion of a patient crowdsourcing her health care causes many a physician's heart to race and breathing to become labored. Before the Internet came along there were already enough snake-oil cures and dangerously misleading health advice out there. Now the floodgates are open.

In the pre-Internet days, health care providers had the comfort of knowing that discerning patients relied on questions to doctors as the primary source of medical knowledge. A few astute consumers also purchased doorstopper-size, hardcover volumes such as The American Medical Association's Family Medical Guide and The Physicians' Desk Reference, which at least carried the imprimatur of medical legitimacy.

Not any more. Anyone with a few rudimentary computer skills and a few bucks can publish a website on a purported miracle cure and say anything he or she likes almost without fear. (An exception, of course, is the Federal Drug Administration's oversight of certain product or treatment health claims.) Heck, you don't even need the few bucks – just find yourself a website with visitor commenting options and say about anything you like.

It's close to impossible to know exactly how many health websites exist. A reasonable guess as any comes from Robert Kiley, London-based editor of the newsletter *He@lth Information on the Internet*, who posits the number at about 100,000.[2]

Regardless, the amount of health information available at the click of the mouse is beyond stupefying. Google counts more than 2.6 million Web pages just on WebMD.com.

2 http://1.usa.gov/MHqnoU

All this points to an immutable reality: health care information, opinion and advice is out there in massive quantities, and people are going to access it regardless of accuracy. For a look at the growing role played by non-physicians in patient decisions, the Pew Research Center did extensive telephone polling of 3,001 adults. In a February 28, 2011, report of its findings,[3] Pew says:

> Seventy percent of American adults say they received information, care or support from a health professional.
>
> Fifty-four percent say they turned to friends and family.
>
> Twenty percent say they turned to others with the same health condition.

"This report shows," Pew concludes, "how people's networks are expanding to include online peers, particularly in the crucible of rare disease."

Connecting online with others through shared interests is called community building. Web 2.0 and social media exist purely due to the power of communities. There are such health websites galore, such as MyLifeline.org, CancerNetwork.com and the ubiquitous WebMD.com, with more than 100 disease group communities.

The numbers on these sites are impressive. Each has a Google PageRank of 5 or higher and an Alexa Ranking below 200,000, putting them in the 99th percentile of all websites on the Internet in terms of popularity. (We look more at these two rankings in the pages ahead.)

More cogently, none of these sites is a pipsqueak. MyLifeline.org is the smallest, at about 1,000 pages. CancerNetwork.com boasts more than 35,000 pages, and WebMD.com is edging toward 3 million pages.

Online medical authority: Who's got it

Amid this profusion of free information online, what's a medical practice to do? Become a Web publisher, too? The answer is resoundingly yes. And it's actually not that hard or expensive.

As difficult as it may be to imagine, small to medium medical practices can swim in this competitive pool by offering useful, patient-oriented health information on their websites. To be sure, no practice is likely to put the resources into winning the Olympics of online health information. But we're not talking about, say, a cardiology group trying to match WebMD.com's 2,000 articles on heart disease, or the 30,000 Web pages on womenshealth.gov if you're an OB/GYN. For most practices, a website with a few dozen pages on specialty-related, patient-oriented health information is plenty enough.

3 http://bit.ly/NuXtdh

A website with 50-100 pages on patient information:

Helps search engines lead more new patients to the site.

Makes the site more interesting, thereby keeping prospective patients on it longer.

Creates an edge over competing practices, many of which publish crudely designed and written sites containing mostly self-interested information.

In the Web world, the term for keeping website visitors longer is making the site stickier. Stickier websites generate more new patients, according to both hard data and observation.

Unfortunately, the majority of medical practice websites are static electronic brochures that are all about doctors and say preciously little about patients and their needs. The conversation starts with seller talk, not customer wants.

The quantity and quality of information on health websites matters a lot to health care consumers because they want authoritative information in one place. Information rules. Patients don't go to doctors just for cures. They go perhaps as much because they want to know. They want knowledge about what might be wrong with them, what might cure it, and whether it might come back.

This book's most important message:

Patients look online for information first and doctors second.

How do I know? Because Google tells me all the time.

The number of searches on Google ranges from 400 billion per day[4] to 1 billion daily.[5] The mighty search engine keeps track of all those searches, and one benefit is that you can get a comparative idea of what people are searching for. Google will tell you in hopes of selling you advertising. Let's look at just a small sample of the topics Google users are searching and in what frequency.

The table on the opposite page is far from representing a scientific sample. Yet for every search for physicians specializing in cancer care (highlighted in italics and light-green boxes), there are **seven times as many searches for the six most common types of cancer.** Even if you look at only the top three most common cancer types, the ratio is still 5.6 to 1.

Granted, patients traditionally have not been as much in the habit of looking online for doctors as they are for, say, where to buy take-out pizza. But that is changing at warp

4 http://bit.ly/NJM4DI

5 http://bit.ly/Ta5B5p

Search terms	Number of Google searches/month
breast cancer	3,350,000
lung cancer	1,220,000
prostate cancer	1,000,000
colorectal cancer	823,000
oncologist	823,000
bladder cancer	301,000
uterine cancer	201,000
cancer doctor	60,500
cancer specialist	33,100

Summary

- *Sample monthly Google searches for information on cancer: 6.9 million*
- *Sample monthly Google searches for information on cancer specialists: 916,660*

speed. For evidence, go to any of a number of business-review and rate-your-doctor websites and see the explosion of patient reviews of their physicians. Examples include Yelp.com, Vitals.com and even Google Maps, where reviews are sourced from other websites (such as Yelp.com) and displayed in Google's search results.

We can also learn much from website analytics, software that tells us how many visitors come to a website and what they see and do there. Web developers have a wide range of choices available for analytics tools, some of which are free, notably Google Analytics.

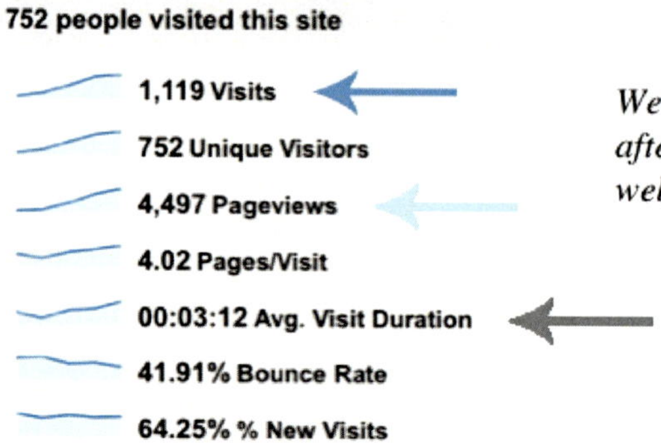
752 people visited this site
1,119 Visits
752 Unique Visitors
4,497 Pageviews
4.02 Pages/Visit
00:03:12 Avg. Visit Duration
41.91% Bounce Rate
64.25% % New Visits

Website metrics for the first month after the launch of a new practice website.

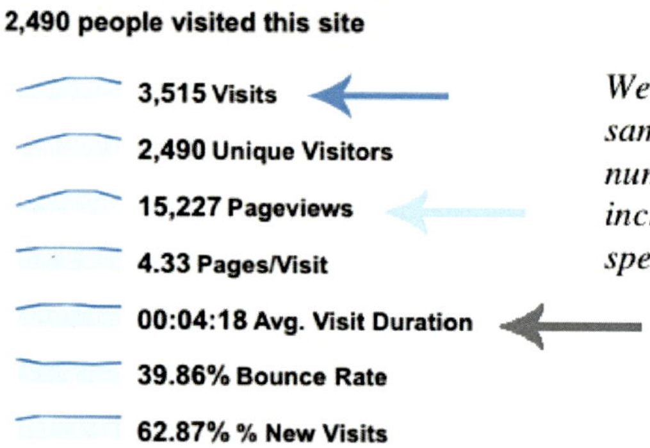
2,490 people visited this site
3,515 Visits
2,490 Unique Visitors
15,227 Pageviews
4.33 Pages/Visit
00:04:18 Avg. Visit Duration
39.86% Bounce Rate
62.87% % New Visits

Website metrics at month six for the same website. Notice a tripling in the number of visits and a 41-percent increase in time the average visitor spent on the website.

Above are data from Google Analytics for month one and month six of a new website for a medical practice. Notice the increases in not only the number of visits to the site but also the amount of time the average visitor spent on the site and the number of pages s/he viewed.

Over this same period, **the amount of patient-oriented information also nearly quadrupled,** rising from 22 pages at launch of the website to 81 pages at month six.

To illustrate this connection between the size of an online site and the quantity and quality of website visits, before and after maps of medical practice's website are on the next page. Web developers typically refer to these diagrams as information architecture (IA) maps, which are organized by link navigation.

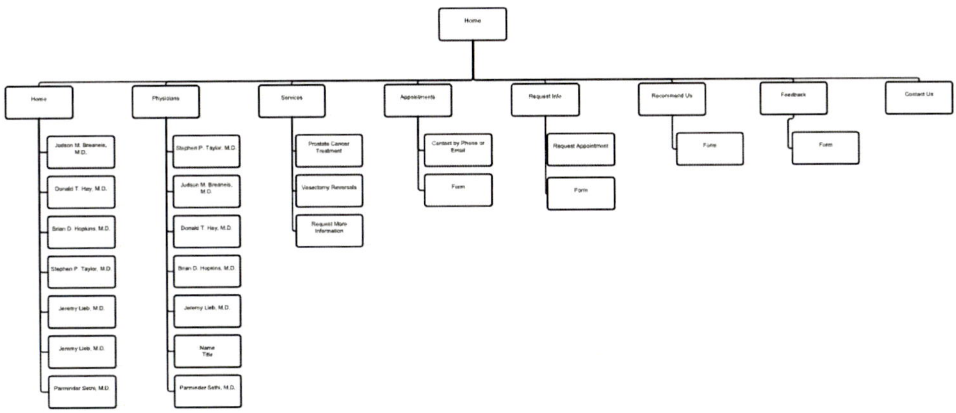
Home
Home
Physicians
Services
Appointments
Request Info
Recommend Us
Feedback
Contact Us
Donald T. Hay, M.D.
Brian D. Hopkins, M.D.
Stephen P. Taylor, M.D.
Jeremy Lieb, M.D.
Parminder Sethi, M.D.
Name
Title
Prostate Cancer Treatment
Vasectomy Reversals
Request More Information
Contact by Phone or Email
Form
Request Appointment
Form
Form
Form

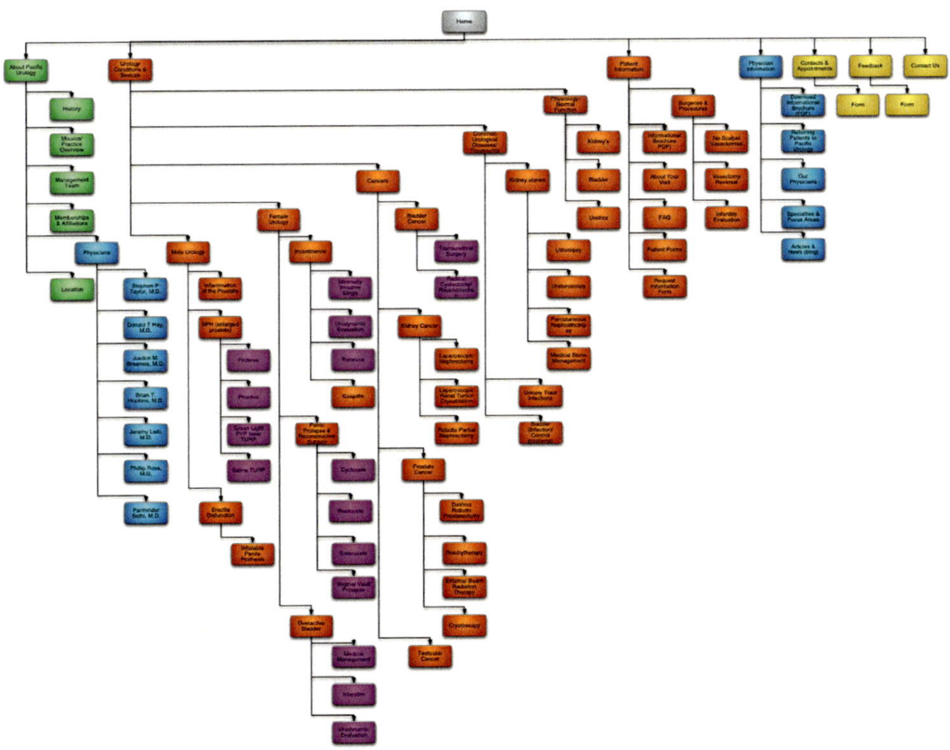

It's easy to notice the shift from physician focus to patient focus. However, for the sake of argument, let's say that it doesn't necessarily occur to the average Internet searcher of cancer information to also look online for cancer physicians. Let's also say that in that searcher's experience, s/he quickly finds an abundance of apparently trustworthy cancer information s/he's looking for and *it's on the website of a nearby medical practice*. What is her likely reaction? It would have to be one or more of the following:

Hey, there's some really good stuff here.

It's interesting that a group of local doctors would go to so much trouble. I'm not even a patient there.

This group of doctors is interested in my learning something.

This group of doctors is trying to lure me into becoming a patient.

From the perspective of the physicians responsible for the website, three of the four possibilities mean the website has made very good first impressions. And even the fourth possibility could mean a good first impression.

The kind of people that doctors want as patients aren't stupid; they're aware that doctors need patients, and they're ready to consider seeing any doctor who generously offers free information with no catches. If all other factors are equal, when it comes time to select a physician, a patient will all but surely favor a doctor or practice offering a profusion of free health information over one who offers little to none.

Easing into patient conversations

In the foreword of this book, I noted that patients don't yet have the luxury of an annual Consumer Reports guide to physicians nationwide. Compared with just about every other purchase available, there is an extraordinary lack of objective evaluations on health care providers available to the public.

What's a patient to do? Well, he's to use the only health care information available to him, which these days generally flows from a combination of sources: a) what his primary care physician tells him, b) what friends and family say about doctors and hospitals and treatments, and c) what he finds online.

Patients have been talking about their health face to face for centuries. Now they have a new medium for it. The Pew Research Center and others have well documented the public swarm toward online health information. This isn't any different from any other topic – does anyone question anymore the cliché that on the Web, content is king?

To earn patients' trust, the easiest first step for health care providers is giving patients what they want: information about their health conditions and possible treatments.

A physician will ultimately be part of every patient's conversation in the exam room and beyond. Why not start the conversation before the patient sets foot in the clinic?

An encyclopedic health care website can form the core of online patient communications and conversations. Moreover, a robust online health library gets the practice in front of more information foragers, as we shall see next.

Chapter 10

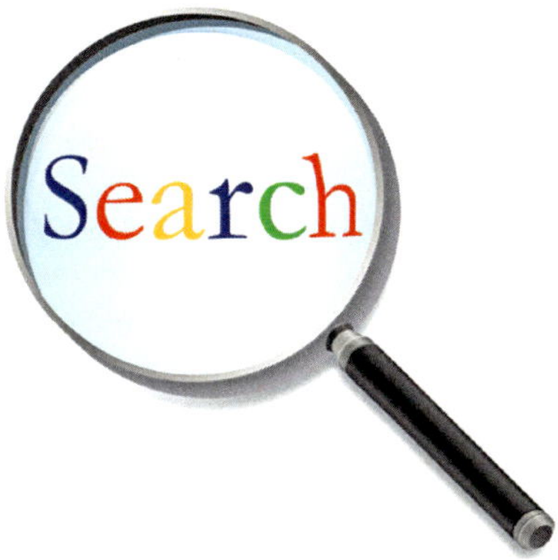

Google is your best friend

& doesn't care about you

SEO as Google owns & controls it

We'll turn our attention now to search-engine optimization (SEO) – a subject that seems to be a popular obsession in recent years – from the perspective of Google, a company with unprecedented impact on humans and commerce the world over.

Google is far from the Internet's only search engine, but it's the one that counts most. From its birth as an obscure 1996 research project of two doctoral students at Stanford University, Google has exploded into the Internet's supernova. The most conservative estimates put Google's share of all Internet searches at around 65 percent. In distant second place are Bing-Yahoo!, two search engines that merged in 2009 and account (by most estimates) for less than 30 percent of Internet searches.[1] Several hundred other search engines are scrapping over the remaining 5 percent or so.

For the most part, whatever Google does is what other search engines do. So at the risk of over-generalization, we'll look how Google works broadly as representative of nearly all search engines.

1 http://ex.pn/PESEKK

But first, an important note: With all its complexities, search engine optimization is not a discipline that most people need to learn. It's a craft best left to technicians. We will not delve into the nuts and bolts here. If you're really interested in the minutiae, there are literally thousands of SEO books on the market. I suggest you pick up one or two and knock yourself out.

Now, back to Google. Valued somewhere north of $100 billion,[2] Google makes mountains of money from advertising. It's critical to grasp this fact fully, as most of what Google does is, by just about every measure, independent of advertising.

Let's take the example of a Google search, using the word "cancer," yielding the search-engine results page (SERP) below.

Search engines give searchers two categories of results: the kind that website publishers have earned and the type they've paid for. **Organic**, or natural searches, appear in the center column of SERPs. These returns are based on secret and proprietary algorithms, extremely complex formulae that assess what a searcher may be truly searching for.

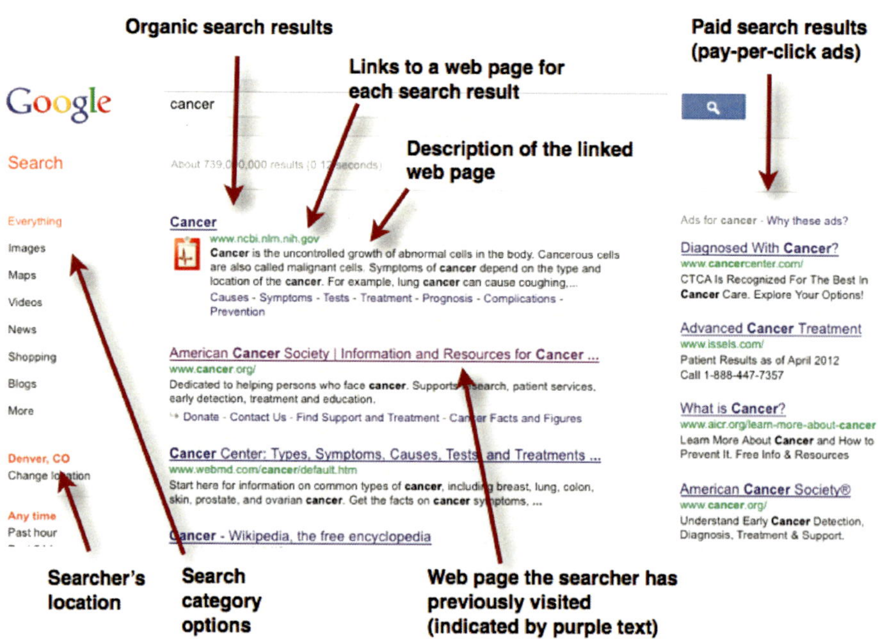

2 http://bloom.bg/ODBbRq

How does Google know, for instance, if a searcher for "hot dogs" is interested in food or very warm puppies? Being able to tell the difference is the beauty of a great search engine. Optimizing a Web page in order to earn high organic rankings is what competent SEO firms do, sometimes for big bucks. It can be very difficult, especially for a term as broad and commonly searched as "cancer" (30.4 million searches a month).

Paid search results are what made the founders of Google (Sergey Brin and Larry Page) stinkin' rich before age 30. These appear in the right column of a SERP and often in the center column, in a faintly yellow box just above the organic returns. These returns are known as pay-per-click (PPC) advertisements because sellers pay for them – but only if and when a Google searcher clicks on the green-text link within the ad and goes to another Web page, known as a *landing page*.

In paid search, the advertiser selects the words in the blue headline, the landing page (indicated by the link below the headline), and the two lines in black text below that, which are each limited to 70 characters maximum. The rankings of these returns are ranked based on two factors: how much each advertiser is willing to spend for click and the rate at which searchers click.

Paid search is wholly distinct from search-engine optimization, a discipline limited exclusively to organic or natural searches. For this reason, we will set aside the topic of PPC ads and devote our attention to organic search for the remainder of this chapter, in hopes of shedding some light via a few myths and facts.

Five great Google myths

Myth one: A search on Google is a live search of the Internet

Here's a reasonably astounding fact: If the Internet crashed tomorrow and took down millions of websites, there would be a backup. Google has a copy of the World Wide Web. So does Bing-Yahoo! and other search engines.

That's right, each major search engine not only has a copy of virtually all websites, but it also updates the copies every second of every day of the year. That's how search engines work.

When you do a search on Google.com, the results aren't gathered directly from the Internet. Instead, you're seeing a snapshot Google took of part of the Internet. The snapshots come from so-called "bots" (tech slang for *robots*) or "spiders" that "crawl" websites. These information-gathering bits of software follow links from Web page to Web page, snagging data on text, still images and videos on each page.

The bots bring it all back to Google's databases that live on a humongous collection of computers all around the world. Here is where Google organizes or "indexes" and stores the data – much like librarians catalog and shelve books according to the Dewey Decimal Classification system developed nearly 150 years ago.

In another library analogy, the information a search engine has about a Web page may not be up to date. Sometimes that information is days, weeks or months old or older, just like an older edition of a book resting on a library shelf. In some cases, the indexed Web page may not even exist any longer, which is why you sometimes get an "Error 404" message when you click on a SERP link. It just means that the publisher of that page took it down since a search-engine bot was last there.

We can easily forgive search engines for such hiccups. Imagine the challenge of staying on top of millions of ever-changing websites. In 2008, Google announced that it had reached the milestone of recording 1 trillion Web addresses (URLs). The truly mind-blowing fact about all major search engines is that they can find, retrieve and display millions of search results in a few tenths of a second. So a very tiny number of results are dead-ends. Big deal. Google's copiously brilliant attributes more than make up for it.

Myth two: SEO rankings can be altered by super geeks & secret technology

Buyer beware – this is the biggest myth of all. The meteoric rise in the number of SEO consultants and firms has created a major industry with far more than its fair share of charlatans. All sizes and shapes of dubious SEO enterprises have sprung up to claim that they have special technology and secret sauces that will catapult your website to the top of organic rankings, as long as you fork over the bucks.

Baloney, hogwash and codswallop.

Go to bookseller Amazon.com and type "search engine optimization" into Amazon's search window. You'll discover in excess of 5,000 books published on the topic, nearly the same as on the subject of plumbing. In comparison, Amazon lists a little more than 4,000 books for sale on French cooking. Ahem. You would thing there would be more secret sauces in French kitchens than in manipulating search rankings.

The truth is that no one knows exactly how Google and other search engines work. The Google algorithm is as much a closely held secret as the formula for Coca-Cola. One reason is clearly proprietary: Google doesn't want imitators trying to steal its business. The other reason is that Google is constantly changing it in order to stay ahead of SEO charlatans trying to game the system.

Nonetheless, tens of thousands of SEO professionals worldwide have a pretty good handle on Google's organic ranking factors. Being effective at SEO is not all that different than being a good doctor, only far less complex and with much lower stakes. A modest amount of study, practice and staying on top of search trends can make a talented SEO technician. You can learn the craft entirely online, if you wish. Three or four years of experience would likely put you in the 90 percentile of SEO whizzes. Secret sauce, my foot.

Myth three: Google is spying on you

Hardly. No doubt, Google is highly interested in its users' habits collectively and stores trillions of bits of data about global usage. It's also interested in your interests and preferences. But it's not tracking you personally, only your computer.

In Part I we covered the topic of Internet protocol (IP) addresses. Every computer on the Internet – including your desktop, laptop and tablet – has an IP number. Google wants to know which computer is conducting searches for both Google's and your own interests. It notes the IP address of each computer for each search.

Sure, Google is doing this because it wants to serve up PPC ads that might lead a searcher to click on one or more and earn it a buck or two. But it also wants to help you with organic search results. That's what will keep you coming back to Google. In this sense, it's no different than a TV network or a magazine – the idea is to keep searchers, viewers and readers interested with relevant entertainment and information in order to sell more advertising.

Google is tracking only your computer by its IP address. Your search habits are going to be mixed in with anyone else using the same computer, whether it's your 87-year-old grandmother or your 13-year-old son.

Myth four: Your website can dominate all Google organic rankings

Unless you're Facebook or YouTube, it's simply not possible in organic rankings, only in pay-per-click ads, and even then often at high cost. For organic rankings, every fiber of Google's being is oriented toward fair play. With few exceptions, no one website can be all things to all Googlers.

Two Google facts are critical:

Google ranks web pages, not websites.

Each page is ranked differently for different search terms (also called keywords).

The latter point is especially important in health care. A page can rank highly for the search term "Los Angeles prostate cancer clinic" but quite poorly for "Los Angeles breast cancer clinic." Both are what SEO specialists call long-tail keywords, with three or more words in each string.

Generally, the longer the search term, the easier it is for Google to find what the searcher is really looking for. (Similarly, in marketing, long-tail searchers are considered more likely to become paying customers.) But notice how the change of one word – from *prostate* to *breast* – makes all the difference medically. It makes just as much of a difference to Google – because it makes all the difference to Google users. In all probability, a searcher interested in one of those words is not going to be at all interested in the other.

In SEO, the rule of thumb is one topic/one Web page. Focus each Web page narrowly, and the Google gods will smile down upon you.

Myth five: Google is eager to right alleged wrongs against you

The hard reality is that Google's not waiting for the phone to ring with complaints from you, not unless you're in the top tier of customers. Remember, Google rakes in more than $40 billion annually, mostly from its advertising sales. That's more than Rupert Murdoch's News Corp. earns.

Google did not succeed because it opened employee-staffed customer-service centers in every neighborhood in America. Rather, the company is a textbook study of computer-driven business efficiencies. A Google sale does not require employee involvement. When a customer buys advertising on Google, he does it all through online automated processes, handing over credit card details, enabling the big, bad G-machine to siphon cash in constant drips until you've spent a bundle before you know it.

Nonetheless, if you spend upward of $10,000 monthly on Google ads, Google will assign an account representative to you. The rep can be quite useful in certain circumstances, although it's nothing like the service you'd get if you hired an accountant or attorney for $10,000 a month.

A co-worker at my firm relates an anecdote from working for a prior employer who was spending approximately $100,000 a month in PPC ads on Google. After a year of expenditures at this rate, Google sent a thank-you gift: a $25 Starbucks gift certificate. In other words, a million bucks got the Google customer a half-dozen free Grande Caramel Macchiatos.

Another anecdote comes from a client practice convinced that Google wrongly double-charged it by tens of thousands of dollars for simultaneous and duplicate PPC campaigns. The practice spent months emailing Google and imploring for a mere telephone call to discuss the issue. The practice never got a response.

In organic search, Google cares even less about how you fare. Does another medical practice in town always rank above you no matter how many SEO consultants you hire? Cry me a river. Not my problem, Google would say.

Five greater Google facts

Fact one: Google wants to help you

As noted earlier, Google lives and dies by how well it matches Internet searchers to relevant information. The techno gorilla spends enormous resources figuring out how to make its search engine the biggest and baddest. Its job is to bring together information searchers and information providers. Period.

Work hard at providing more information and Google will bring you more searchers. We've seen medical practice websites double, triple and even quadruple their visits in short order as a result of adding online health information. We've also seen the same websites rocket upward in search rankings. The two results go together, side by side.

Fact two: Unlike teens, Google pays highest respect to age & wisdom

Search engines give much heed to both the volume of content on a Web page and the age of the Web page's root URL (i.e., the home page address). All things equal, a practice with a 10-year-old URL will place better in Google rankings than a practice with a brand-new URL.

In a similar vein, Google respects smart Web pages. Aside from its own sophisticated algorithm, Google measures smartness by popular opinion. Actually, there's a historical anecdote that might be of interest to physicians and scientists.

In the early days of developing their search engine at Stanford, Page and Brin made the case that an Internet search tool should pattern scientific literature and journals. That is, research papers with the most citations in subsequent research papers must be the most important work. This is one definition of seminal research.

Following this concept, websites with the most inbound links from other websites covering the same topics must therefore be of the highest value. Back-linking therefore played a major role in the algorithm of Page and Brin's prototype search engine, which they initially named BackRub, for obvious reasons.

Today, inbound links still matter a lot to Google and search engines. Most SEO specialists agree that the quantity and quality of back links are the single most important factor in search rankings.

Fact three: Google likes reputation, clarity & usability equally

What is building quality inbound links to a website all about? It's about providing not just thorough and useful information, but also well-organized information.

If they're smart, publishers of other websites pick and choose carefully where they wish to send their own visitors. It takes a lot to fetch visitors to your site. Why surrender them to another site easily?

Attracting the attention of other websites requires careful organization and structure of your own website. This includes a well-planned site navigation structure. Sure, it's terrific to have sizable site, but you lose some of the advantages if visitors are constantly going down blind alleys on your website and can't find their way around.

Don't take just my word for it. Here's how one SEO firm views it:

> *Size only matters when used properly. Empty pages with no authority are of no help to SEO. What is important to size and search is creating as many* ***quality authoritative*** *pages as possible. Some of the keys to building page authority are: 1) Building quality inbound links, 2) Creating effective internal pathways to your pages, 3) Providing quality unique content on each important page of your website*

Have you noticed how most hospitals end up growing into a convoluted maze of hallways and corridors? With time, growing websites also tend to sprawl out of control in the same manner. A good website is never actually finished. There's always more information to publish online. As your practice's website grows, be careful to avoid a website as disorienting as your local hospital.

Fact four: Google pays close attention to each searcher's location

You may have heard the axiom that Internet search is increasingly local. It's true. Particularly with the boom in smart phones, Google is extremely intent on knowing the precise location of each searcher. If you're looking on Google for Chinese food, it stands to reason that Google prefers to send you to websites of Chinese restaurants a few minutes' drive away, rather than halfway across the country.

The same is true for desktop, laptop and tablet computers that don't use cell phone technology to connect with Google. In such cases, each computer connects to the Internet through a modem, which also has an IP address. Internet service providers such as telephone and cable-TV companies assign IP addresses to modems based on the modem's location.

For this reason, a search for mechanics or dentists or cardiologists will yield different results in different cities. This is how it's possible for a practice's website to rank highly among local searchers. Otherwise, every cardiology group's website would be completely lost in the rankings to, say, the American Heart Association or the Mayo Clinic's voluminous section on heart health.

Fact five: Google isn't going to crown you king anytime soon

A frequent complaint from customers of SEO consultants and firms is that after six, 12 or 24 months, their website still isn't top of the mountain in search results. Doggone it, the websites of the American Heart Association, the Mayo Clinic, WebMD and Wikipedia still dominate page one of SERPs for short-tail search terms such as *heart disease*.

Get used to the fact that this won't change, probably ever. Such organizations have worked their way to the top of the heap online and offline. An organization of several dozen employees isn't going to knock them off the pedestal.

But you can make steady progress upward, especially against competing practices. Keep in mind that Internet search gets increasingly local all the time. Furthermore, the most qualified prospective patients use long-tail keywords. For example, there's a huge difference in page one of SERPs between the keyword *heart disease* and *heart disease Dallas*.

The latter keyword set is what's called geo-targeted, and as I write this, it results in a first-place organic Google ranking for a Dallas cardiology practice. Nice work, Dallas cardiologists. But don't rest on your laurels. Another practice could pass you.

Keeping the information warehouse fully stocked

At the end of the day, the lesson is that the best never rest. If you're part of managing a medical practice, you can't go wrong thinking of your website as one of the clinic locations that deserves ongoing attention. It's a virtual clinic, where no one can physically show up but many can attend electronically.

If you've done a good job of being an online resource to both current and prospective patients alike, and Google has responded appropriately, chances are better than 50-50 that your website's analytics will reveal an astounding fact:

> *An educational, patient-centric website will bring more visits in a month than any of a medical practice's clinic locations.*

That's correct, month in and month out, more people will see the practice website than the inside of your offices, sometimes by a multiple. This is even more the case if you continue to update the website with fresh and timely information.

As information shoppers, health care consumers like to browse websites with a wealth of up-to-date inventory. Correspondingly, search engines reward the department-store equivalent on the Web by bringing larger crowds to peruse the information merchandise. Larger and more informative websites make a bigger target for search engines and visitors.

Give health care consumers new reasons to find your website and keep coming back to it. Otherwise, as the saying goes, if you rest you'll rust.

Chapter 11

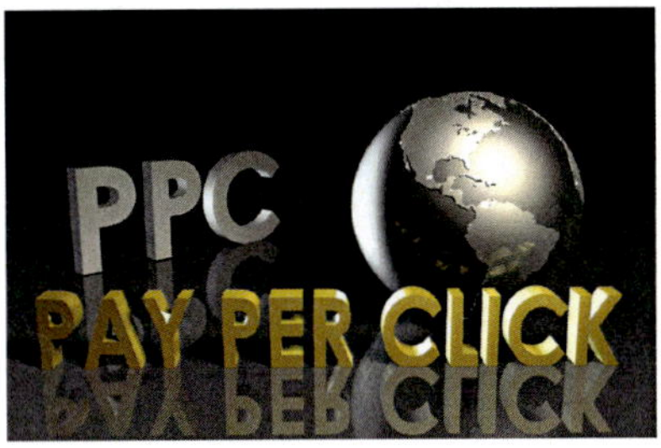

Advertising on the Internet

Sponsored search-engine ads & pay-per-click truths

Okay, students of medical marketing, let's see who can answer this easy question: How many of you have ever shopped for a car dealer? What? None of you? No, of course not. People shop for cars, not car dealers.

Yes, eventually car buyers wind up transacting with a dealer, but only because if they want a new car, they are all but forced to purchase from a manufacturer-authorized dealer – even if it's an online dealer or car-buying service.

If you've been watching the social data the last few years, it's clear the same mind-set has been creeping into doctor shopping. To be sure, a physician-patient relationship is a long ways from the often barely tolerable hour or so you spend with a car salesman every few years. Patients are typically more discerning about the professional and personal traits of their health care providers than they are about their clergy, bankers, accountants or any other service professional.

Yet for millions of Americans today, picking a doctor starts not with a search for a health care provider but a search for health care information. But more important is an unmistakable trend in who patients are asking to provide such information.

This trend is precisely why medical practices should be soberly realistic about the value of pay-per-click advertising on search engines.

PPC ads: A clandestine auction

For those new to the PPC concept of marketing, here's how it works: You the seller may offer your products or services for sale on the pages of search-engine websites. Internet searchers using Google, Yahoo! and Bing see these on almost every query result, under a "sponsored links" heading in search-engine results pages (SERP).

These sponsored links are always limited to two lines of text, 130 characters total, with a hyperlink to the advertiser's website on a third line. PPC adds appear above and to the right of the rest of the listings on the SERP, which are known as "organic" or "natural" search-engine results.

PPC ads are also often presented on a pastel background on the SERP. However, one disturbing search-engine trend has been to lessen the contrast between PPC ads and organic listings, blurring the differences between paid advertising and organic rankings – the latter depending on a relatively fair methodology of ranking Web pages based on how well their content relates to what Internet searchers are seeking.

PPC advertisers select certain search phrases to trigger displays of their ads. For example, a car dealer might select "Phoenix Honda dealers" or "2011 Accord pricing" as terms that cause the dealer's PPC ad to appear each time a Google user types those words (or some of those words) into the Google search engine.

PPC ads are what make Google so staggeringly successful, earning the company more than $30 billion a year. One reason is that this form of marketing is truly revolutionary. Unlike traditional advertising in newspapers, magazines and on billboards, radio and TV, PPC advertisers don't pay just to have their ads displayed. The display of an ad – or an impression – is free. Rather, the advertiser pays Google or Bing or whomever only each time someone clicks on one of their ads – hence, the pay-per-click nomenclature.

Why click-through rates rule

Another reason for PPC success for Google et al is the unique pricing system. PPC advertisers bid for positioning. The more you offer to pay for a clicker coming from Google to your website, generally the higher your ad ranks on SERPs.

But wait, there's another sizable factor in PPC ad ranking: popularity. Ranking of your ad also depends on the percentage of Google users clicking on the ad. This is called the "click through rate." The CTR is calculated by dividing the number of clicks on an ad by the number of times it was displayed.

Thus, if your PPC ad is displayed 10,000 times in response to certain search phrases being entered into a search engine, and 500 of those times someone clicks on your ad, your CTR is 5 percent – a rather high CTR, given that 1 or 2 percent CTR is far more common.

The kicker: you don't know how much other advertisers are bidding in competition against you. You can only make an educated guess at how much to bid and hope your ad ranks relatively high. Bidding usually begins at 15 cents per click, and can range up to $10 or more, depending on the value of the search term you're bidding on, the demand for the product or service you're selling, and other factors. Some heath care search terms fetch $10 or more for top-ranking positions.

Over time, Google or the search engine you the PPC advertiser is using will tell you how well each ad is ranking in the PPC listings. The trick is to manage the search terms, the bidding, and the ad text so that you get maximum CTR for the lowest possible price.

Because more clicks mean more income to Google, the search engine likes to see your CTR rise and will reward you by increasing your rankings without charging more.

Whew, sounds like a lot of work, right? Well, it is. And the bummer is that it can all be for naught, especially in health care.

Selling horseshoes in Times Square

When PPC works, it brings a lot of people to a website. Then what? Can you count on an automatic sale? Hardly.

Growing a medical practice is all about cultivating physician-patient relationships. This personal connection can and should start on a website. But it's not the same as selling to a customer who already knows what she wants to buy and is simply using the Internet to find the best price.

Therefore, you can spend a lot of time and money on PPC advertising and ultimately bring a lot of people to a website, only to have a lot of them look at one or two pages on the site and leave in a matter of seconds. No sale.

It's like opening a horseshoeing service in Times Square. You can have one of the world's busiest locations, but passing crowds don't automatically translate into sales.

By most estimates, less than 10 percent of website visits are generated by PPC ads. That means nine in 10 visits to your practice's website will come through other means, usually by organic searches.

In the end, what really matters is a rich patient experience. Your practice website should be an attractive and fetching store that invites lots of people to come in and browse. It's not merely enough to bring prospective customers only to the front door. The delicate process of nurturing a physician-patient relationship must start with the patient enjoying a prolonged and rewarding experience on multiple pages of the website.

If you don't have such a store on the Internet, forget PPC advertising. You'll wind up paying Times Square prices for a barn no horse will likely enter.

Chapter 12

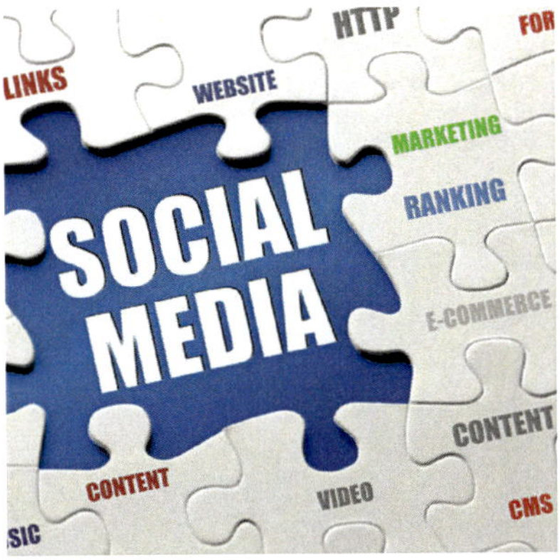

Social media & online reputation management

Facebook: Constructive juggernaut or pointless distraction?

Has the Facebook bug bitten you yet? It's hard not to be infected by the explosive buzz around Facebook's stunning popularity, and to ponder its implications for medicine. First, Hollywood releases a zippy-dialogue movie about Facebook founder Mark Zuckerberg. Then the flick cleans up at the Golden Globe and Academy Awards, winning seven trophies total. Then, Experian Hitwise proclaims the search term "Facebook" to be the most popular on the Internet and Facebook to the most visited website on Earth, nudging ahead of juggernaut Google in popularity.

All the hoopla raises two potentially conflicting questions: Does Facebook have anything to do with patients and doctors, and can anyone afford to ignore it?

The answers are yes and no, respectively.

Today, Facebook accounts for nearly one in 10 visits to websites among Americans. Given the site's popularity, any manager or shareholder in a specialty medical practice might be inclined to say, "If we want more patients, we'd better do something big on Facebook and quick!"

Yes, you should do *something*, although Facebook is not the best place to pour the bulk of your marketing efforts – at least not according to the data my firm has gathered on behalf of medical practices coast to coast. While medical practices should not dismiss Facebook entirely, there are growing signs that other social platforms are having as much or more direct impact on how patients select doctors.

At my medical marketing firm, we manage and make regular postings to both Facebook and Twitter every week. Reality check: We also monitor the source of all visitors to each client medical practice's website. In the best of circumstances – those practices who have the most Facebook followers and Facebook activity – no more than 2 to 3 percent of visits to the practice's website come directly from Facebook.

But let's not be too hasty in calling it a waste of time. By several other measures, Facebook is still an important part of the marketing mix.

The virus you want to catch

With more than 800 million Facebook users, there can be no doubt the prospective pool of patients is present and talking on Facebook in force. Facebook provides precise counts of visits to a practice's Facebook account (called a Page) by day, by week, by month. Facebook also reports the total number of Facebook connections of those visitors. These connections are the heart of social media – as soon as you become a "fan" of a Page, you can post a comment, you can "like" (i.e., endorse) someone else's comment, and you can "share" someone else's posting of a comment (a picture, a video or a link to another Web page) on the Page.

The link in the Page's Facebook posting is a vital component. The whole idea is to bring as many visitors to a practice's website – its virtual clinic – as possible.

In any case, each action on Facebook is noted on the action-taker's "news feed" – all the people with whom you've become Facebook friends are notified of the action. Additionally, whenever you post to your "wall" – a page on your Facebook account where you can initiate your own conversations – that comment also appears on the home pages of all your friends on Facebook.

In other words, Facebook spreads water-cooler talk across the Internet universe in a big, special and ultra-fast way. Every time you sneeze on Facebook, a lot of other people catch your cold. The busy medical practice could choose to ignore those millions of sneezes, but why not help spread the virus instead?

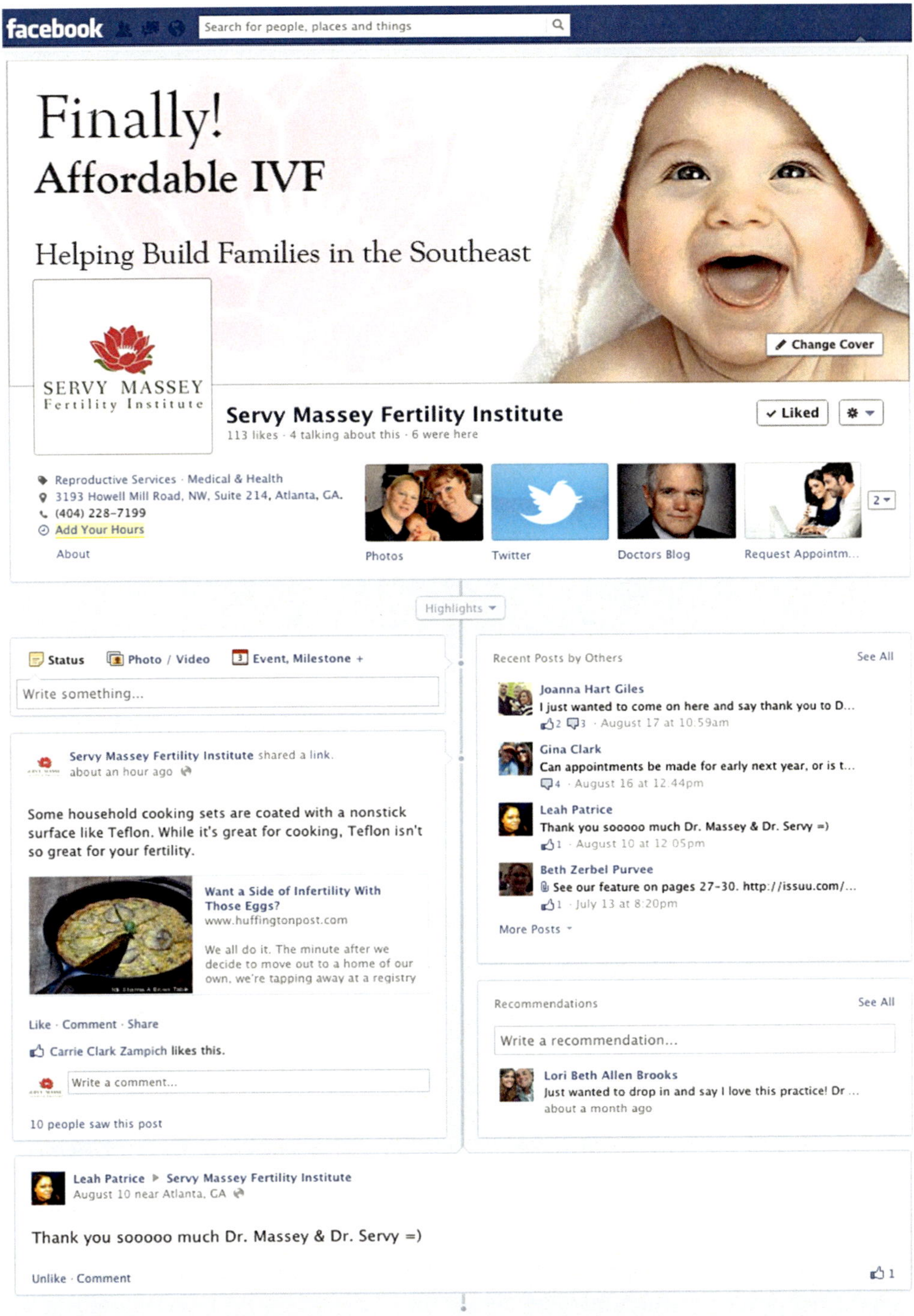
facebook
Search for people, places and things
Finally!
Affordable IVF
Helping Build Families in the Southeast
SERVY MASSEY
Fertility Institute
Change Cover
Servy Massey Fertility Institute
113 likes · 4 talking about this · 6 were here
Liked
Reproductive Services · Medical & Health
3193 Howell Mill Road, NW, Suite 214, Atlanta, GA.
(404) 228-7199
Add Your Hours
About
Photos
Twitter
Doctors Blog
Request Appointm...
Highlights
Status
Photo / Video
Event, Milestone +
Write something...
Servy Massey Fertility Institute shared a link.
about an hour ago
Some household cooking sets are coated with a nonstick surface like Teflon. While it's great for cooking, Teflon isn't so great for your fertility.
Want a Side of Infertility With Those Eggs?
www.huffingtonpost.com
We all do it. The minute after we decide to move out to a home of our own, we're tapping away at a registry
Like · Comment · Share
Carrie Clark Zampich likes this.
Write a comment...
10 people saw this post
Recent Posts by Others
See All
Joanna Hart Giles
I just wanted to come on here and say thank you to D...
2 3 · August 17 at 10:59am
Gina Clark
Can appointments be made for early next year, or is t...
4 · August 16 at 12:44pm
Leah Patrice
Thank you sooooo much Dr. Massey & Dr. Servy =)
1 · August 10 at 12:05pm
Beth Zerbel Purvee
See our feature on pages 27-30. http://issuu.com/...
1 · July 13 at 8:20pm
More Posts
Recommendations
See All
Write a recommendation...
Lori Beth Allen Brooks
Just wanted to drop in and say I love this practice! Dr ...
about a month ago
Leah Patrice ▸ Servy Massey Fertility Institute
August 10 near Atlanta, GA
Thank you sooooo much Dr. Massey & Dr. Servy =)
Unlike · Comment
1

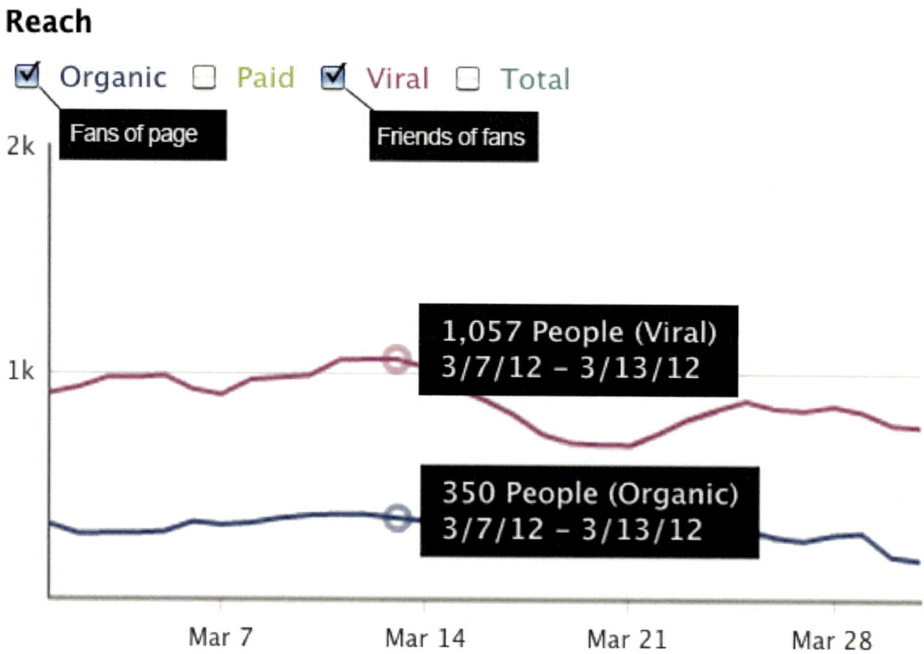

The idea, then, is to have just a few patients – you don't need a lot in order to have a nice impact – say a few special words about their doctors on Facebook. Based on our analysis of Facebook, each posting on a medical practice's Page has the potential to reach a lot of people. This sample "Reach" graph shows with one posting on March 7, 2012, a total of 1,407 Facebook users were reached that week.

This leads the reasonable person to conclude that the discerning doctor shopper may well visit Facebook just to see what kind of presence any physician or practice may have there. It just makes sense that a significant number of prospective patients will check out a doctor or a practice on Facebook to see what others are saying about the practice, if anything.

If a Page has a few more "likes" and interactions from happy patients than their competitors, that goes a long way toward tilting the prospective patient away from the competitors and toward that practice. You can bet a fair number of Facebookers will compare such data among competing practices (see graphic on following page).

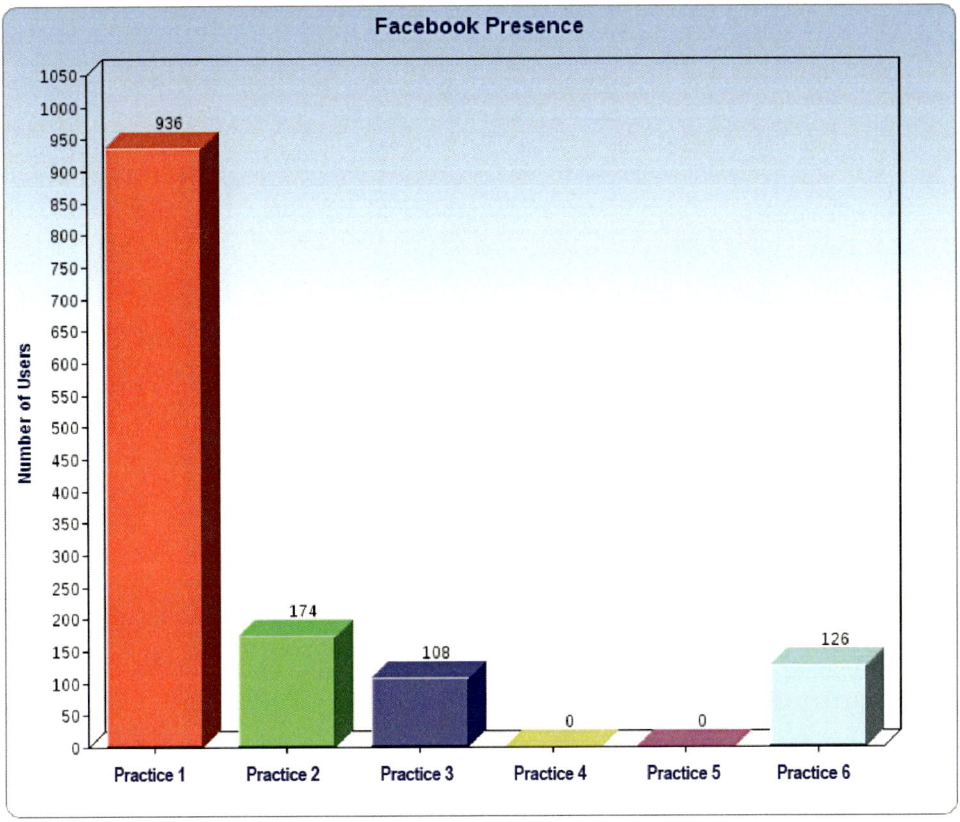

It's quality marketing versus quantity, a common theme of this book. Opening and maintaining multiple lines of new-media communication lets you catch the giant wave of conversation as the most effective marketing tool available, happening live, right now.

In all honesty, we're not talking about hiring a full-time social media employee or consultant to stuff social media sites with practice propaganda – this would be counter-productive. Even making two Facebook postings a month could put your practice well ahead of the competition and be the eventual tiebreaker among a significant number of prospective patients.

Remember, shouting to the wrong crowd – no matter how large – may get you nothing, while whispering to just one person may get you everything.

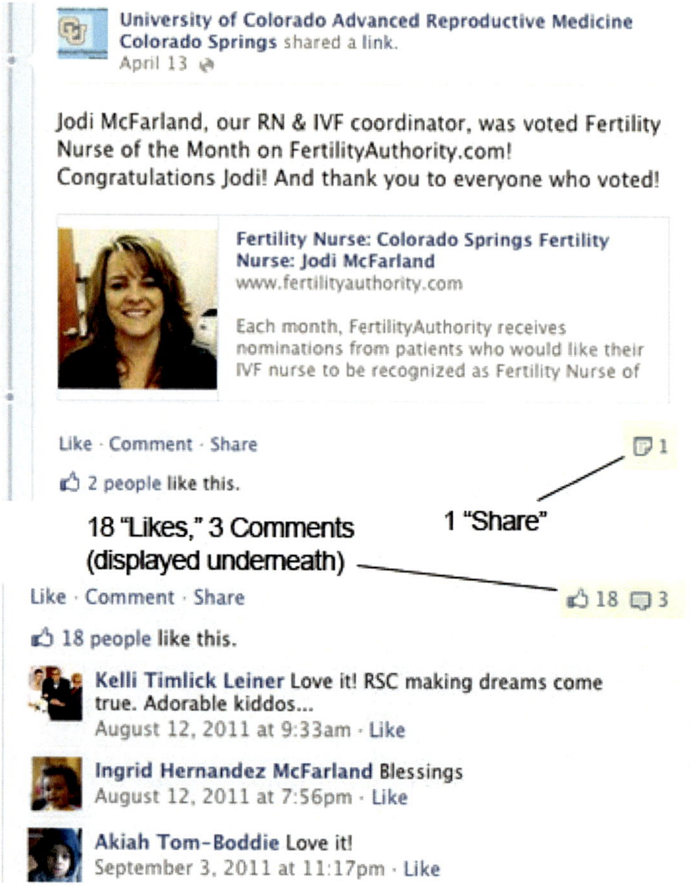
University of Colorado Advanced Reproductive Medicine Colorado Springs shared a link.
April 13
Jodi McFarland, our RN & IVF coordinator, was voted Fertility Nurse of the Month on FertilityAuthority.com! Congratulations Jodi! And thank you to everyone who voted!
Fertility Nurse: Colorado Springs Fertility Nurse: Jodi McFarland
www.fertilityauthority.com
Each month, FertilityAuthority receives nominations from patients who would like their IVF nurse to be recognized as Fertility Nurse of
Like · Comment · Share
1
2 people like this.
18 "Likes," 3 Comments (displayed underneath)
1 "Share"
Like · Comment · Share
18 3
18 people like this.
Kelli Timlick Leiner Love it! RSC making dreams come true. Adorable kiddos...
August 12, 2011 at 9:33am · Like
Ingrid Hernandez McFarland Blessings
August 12, 2011 at 7:56pm · Like
Akiah Tom-Boddie Love it!
September 3, 2011 at 11:17pm · Like

Content rules...again

Facebook – like other social media websites such as Twitter, Google+, and others – is not the place for a hard sell. Participants in the online social sphere are expected to contribute value to their fellow community members through posts and interaction. In other words, no one wants to read an advertisement stuffed into a Facebook post.

This is tempting for specialty medical practices and other businesses alike because distributing a practice's information on Facebook is, of course, free (unless you employ audience-targeted Facebook advertising, which is a whole different animal). Here's the catch: The more you direct attention to a brand via its Facebook page, the more its fans and followers choose not to listen.

To achieve a devoted following, you have to distribute quality content your followers will find beneficial – which generally means not the self-promoting kind. Again, the talk should be less about the seller (the practice) and more about the buyer (the patient).

Think in terms of news stories, community events, photos, and other interesting tidbits fans (patients) might like. The gain is that if fans like what's being posted, they'll be more apt to "like" it, comment on it, or better yet – share it. This in turn, will hopefully gain a bigger following, which means more interaction and engagement, and the circle goes ever on and on.A modest but ever-active Facebook presence strengthens a practice's competitive edge and builds an authoritative reputation, albeit with limited power in comparison to other online efforts. You could think of it this way: Branding and a smart allocation of noise-making tools form the strong arm in building the practice's business, and Facebook is one of the fingers. In some cases, it may be the whisper that tips the scales in winning over a new patient.

Tweets as health conversation starters

Like Facebook, Twitter has become one of the pillars of social media, although with its own flavorings. With around 500 million users, Twitter is the ninth-most popular website on the Internet, according to the technology company Alexa. Its success in tandem with Facebook's meteoric rise is due to its place in many ways as a complement to Facebook rather than always a direct rival.

Twitter limits its postings (called "tweets") to 140 characters, earning it a distinction as a so-called microblog. For this reason, Twitter's stream is somewhat better suited for mobile devices (cell phones and tablet computers). Accordingly, strong calls to action, news blips, and a shortened URL for links is the name of the game for Twitter movers and shakers.

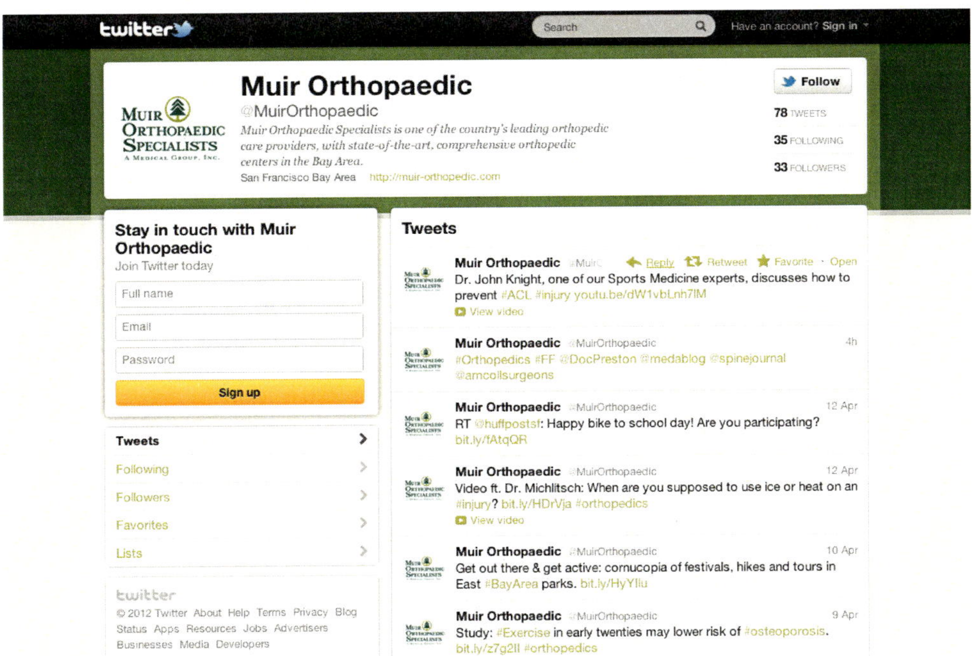
twitter
Search
Have an account? Sign in
Muir Orthopaedic
@MuirOrthopaedic
Muir Orthopaedic Specialists is one of the country's leading orthopedic care providers, with state-of-the-art, comprehensive orthopedic centers in the Bay Area.
San Francisco Bay Area http://muir-orthopedic.com
Muir Orthopaedic Specialists
Follow
78 TWEETS
35 FOLLOWING
33 FOLLOWERS
Stay in touch with Muir Orthopaedic
Join Twitter today
Full name
Email
Password
Sign up
Tweets
Following
Followers
Favorites
Lists
twitter
© 2012 Twitter About Help Terms Privacy Blog
Status Apps Resources Jobs Advertisers
Businesses Media Developers
Tweets
Muir Orthopaedic Reply Retweet Favorite · Open
Dr. John Knight, one of our Sports Medicine experts, discusses how to prevent #ACL #injury youtu.be/dW1vbLnh7IM
View video
Muir Orthopaedic @MuirOrthopaedic 4h
#Orthopedics #FF @DocPreston @medablog @spinejournal @amcollsurgeons
Muir Orthopaedic @MuirOrthopaedic 12 Apr
RT @huffpostsf: Happy bike to school day! Are you participating? bit.ly/IAtqQR
Muir Orthopaedic @MuirOrthopaedic 12 Apr
Video ft. Dr. Michlitsch: When are you supposed to use ice or heat on an #injury? bit.ly/HDrVja #orthopedics
View video
Muir Orthopaedic @MuirOrthopaedic 10 Apr
Get out there & get active: cornucopia of festivals, hikes and tours in East #BayArea parks. bit.ly/HyYIiu
Muir Orthopaedic @MuirOrthopaedic 9 Apr
Study: #Exercise in early twenties may lower risk of #osteoporosis. bit.ly/z7g2Il #orthopedics

Twitter works when there's something to announce – like a new blog post on your website, a service special or other timely news. Keeping abreast and alerting followers to new developments in your practice's field is another way to contribute value to users who subscribe to a business' Twitter feed.

Twitter is another social media tool that helps establish a medical practice as an authority in its field. While Facebook is all about networking with the patients, Twitter is a combination of business-to-consumer (B2C) and business-to-business (B2B) marketing. Who you follow, and who follows you, determines who might prospectively see your tweets, and who might recommend you to their own flock.

But also like Facebook, this isn't the place to herald a practice's greatness ad nauseum. Rather, it's a venue to add your 2 cents and carve a niche in a target community as someone in the know. It's entirely up to the community to become followers of your tweets, although Twitter users are seeking information and if that's what you're offering, they just might take notice.

For businesses, each tweet on Twitter acts as a breadcrumb to tantalize and lead the readers to look into something further. It's then up to the rest of the marketing efforts – such as a blog or website – to really deliver what the searching patient is looking for via well-strategized linking. The 140-character tweet acts as the spark – a headline and conversation starter, with a link to a page on the practice's website as often as not.

Hashing out the trends

What are patients talking about on Twitter? A unique feature of Twitter is that users may still see your content, even if they aren't following the practice's Twitter account.

Hashtags (the "#" sign) are Twitter's way of categorizing and identifying trends among the millions of tweets in the Twittersphere. Topics such as #IVF, #Sports and #Health merge with brand trends like #CocaCola and #Sony. Any Twitter user can search the network's gigantic database of past tweets for these hashtag topics and find new Twitter profiles that they may choose to follow or just choose to pursue the breadcrumbs to the larger source of information.

If played right, Twitter connects prospective patients to the practice's website – and, ideally, a physicians' blog – where the practice's expertise and informational outreach becomes a compelling reason to become a patient.

Blogging as the headwaters of social media

The strongest business case for certain social media efforts is based on an old saying: the more you tell, the more you sell.

Earlier, we noted that the first rule of marketing is to make the choice clear. As a leader in a medical practice, you want a prospective patient to think that your practice and physicians stand out from all others. Maintaining a blog on your practice's website can be the origins of an effective differentiator in a local medical market.

It's a great paradox that the doctors who profit most are those who offer their expertise for free. How else to explain the expanding empires of Drs. Chopra, Oz, Weil and a host of other TV, radio and newspaper docs?

With a website, you don't need a TV show or newspaper column to capitalize on the same opportunities. A free blog written in turns by physicians, nurse practitioners and other clinicians will do just fine. Here are a few practical and business benefits.

Blogging benefit #1: One-to-many communications

We are all acutely aware of how much time clinicians spend in exam rooms answering the same questions posed by multiple patients. A blog can be an excellent shortcut by providing much of the basic clinical information through one-to-many conversations.

In the 21st century, patients increasingly don't begin their treatment in a doctor's office. The groundbreaking work of the Pew Research Center has shown that today's patients begin treatment on the Web, seeking health care information first and then seeking a health care provider as the second step.

The Internet is nothing if not an immensely powerful and efficient tool of information dissemination. Let it enable clinicians to devote more time to healing by answering questions outside the clinic.

Blogging benefit #2: Sorting hope from hype

Anyone in health care is fully aware that press releases about promising medical research – typically funded by pharmaceutical companies – can be as much about commercial hype as realistic hope. In this vein, a client physician once expressed strong reluctance to blog about the so-called "cancer vaccine," an anti-cancer medication in a limited clinical trial.

"There are so many hurdles for this drug to clear that it's unlikely that these treatments will ever hit the market," he said. "Why get people's hopes up?

I would agree that he was half right. Why, indeed, lead cancer patients down a primrose path to a dead-end of disappointment?

The half-wrong part, however, is that his point is actually an argument FOR physicians to blog about these kinds of public proclamations of medical breakthroughs. Put it into this context: right after the cancer-vaccine news broke, if you did a Google search for the commercial name for the drug in trials, you'd get approximately a half-million results.

Two months prior to the news, I'd bet it was not even 5 percent of that. The search results are overt evidence that masses of people are already talking about a cancer vaccine and looking for more related information on the Internet.

In this instance, if you're a physician in private practice – especially in the specialty of urology or oncology – you can either be in on the searches and related public conversations, or out of them altogether.

In the latter case I'd say you're inviting physicians in competing practices to take the opportunity away from you. By no means do people – especially cancer patients – want deception about their diseases. Yes, they want hope and to believe in the best possible outcomes for their treatments. But most of all, they want an authoritative source they can trust.

That would be doctors. Second only to cures for their diseases, what patients want desperately is useful, actionable information. Such information – in various forms of usefulness and accuracy – is already all over the Internet. A blog is a fast and easy way to add your voice of reason to the cornucopia of online opinion.

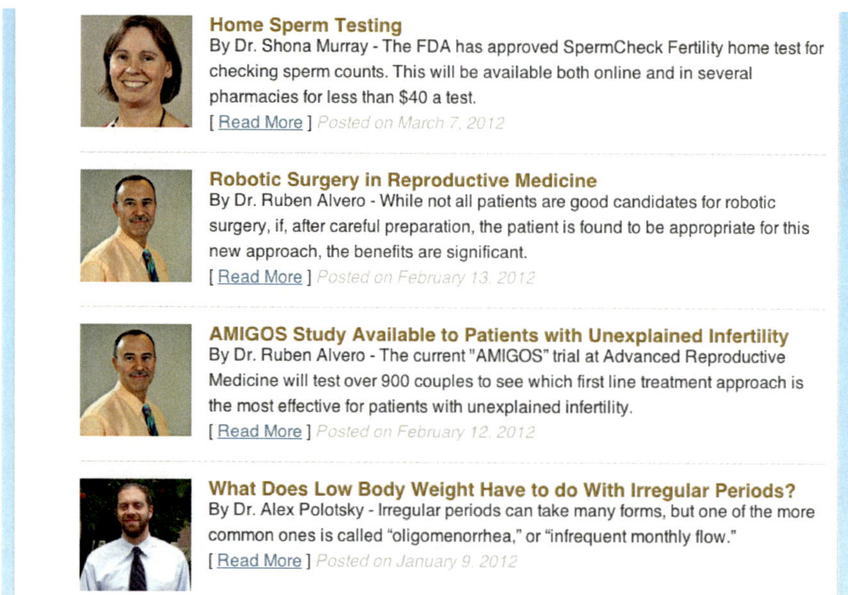

Blogging benefit #3: Steering online conversations

Now we arrive at perhaps the most compelling feature of blogging, the role it can play in influencing online patient conversations. The majority of posts on social media are reactive rather than proactive. Social media users love to go off on one thing or another they've seen on TV or newspapers or websites or somewhere else.

Facebookers, Tweeters et al have a good reason to be more reactive than proactive: it takes less time. Let someone else state their case first. Then you can spout off with far less work than formulating your thoughts in a vacuum.

The evident opportunity for health care experts is to give 'em something to talk about. A blog is an unbeatable conversation starter in the social media space, calling more attention to whoever started the conversation than anyone else. A single blog can spur a half-dozen or more Facebook posts or tweets, feeding the social media monster with no particular time limit imposed.

Physician blogging guidelines

1. Pick a hot topic

Now that you've no doubt been convinced to jump on the blogging bandwagon, following are a few ideas on making it as efficient an exercise as possible.

Patients don't read and don't care about scientific literature. Ninety percent have never heard of the specialty journals their sub-specialty doctors read. Rather, patients search the Web, watch TV, listen to the radio and read newspapers and magazines.

A simple shortcut for picking a blog topic: search Google News or news websites for what's making headlines. Google terms relevant to a practice's specialty on any of these sites and see what comes up. It's guaranteed you'll find some button-pushing topic on which you can barely refrain from commenting.

Chances are good a movie star or sports celebrity may be involved in the news making. All the better. A show business connection generates patient buzz, and you want to opine about what's hot.

2. Keep it short, simple & opinionated

Blogging is counter-intuitive to medical training. It's more about opinions than raw data. Folks out on the Internet like it when the blogger takes a stand.

Of course, a good blogger's opinions ideally should be based on clinical or research evidence. But the idea is to stake out a position. Don't hold back on the newest study or a purported miracle cure or the latest pop-health trend. Tell them exactly what you think, and don't candy-coat it.

Keep your focus on one main point and don't stray to side issues. Six hundred words are about the limit on what you should say, but four hundred words or less are even better.

3. Offer a call to action

Patients don't just want information. They want to know what to do with information. Give them a loose plan, a course of action, and the best possible response to the health consumer's question, "Well, what do I do now?"

Mind you, this isn't to say that you should dispense personalized medical advice in your blog. Steer way clear of ethical and legal liabilities and all the complexities of individual symptoms and circumstances.

Nonetheless, a clinician can make broad but quite useful suggestions, which often fall into the simple advice of something like: "Find a specialist and then ask him or her these kinds of questions." You can also give them the three or four most common options for a certain condition or set of symptoms while closing with the time-proven qualifier: "Of course, it's imperative to see a specialist before you do anything."

Lastly, remember that writer's block is a common disease, affecting even the world's greatest authors. Don't be intimidated by the notion of writing for public consumption. Apply these three guidelines and chances are quite good that your literary stage fright will give way to unbridled expression – and, if you're lucky, a devoted and regular readership.

Online reputation management for doctors

To understand the power of social media in the health care world, let's review a fundamental truth: patients have limited objective ability to judge a physician's skills.

As noted, Consumer Reports sells out its special April automotive issue, while there is no CR equivalent for doctor reviews. As for the annual "Top Doctors" issues of city magazines, the health care consumer receives dubious benefit. Fellow physicians vote on top docs based largely on hearsay, leaving those left out grumbling about a selection process that's as evidence based as the election of prom king and queen.

In a perfect world where the consumer rules all, patients might expect state and local medical societies and specialty associations to furnish comparative data about physician members. Yet many such organizations would sooner spread the Ebola virus than distribute any such information.

Okay, so why not the government as such a purveyor? The National Institutes of Health and the Centers for Disease Control and Prevention publish millions of pages for health care consumers on the Web about virtually all health conditions and treatments known to humans. Why shouldn't they do the same for health care providers?

Well, they do – but only for fertility clinics. Of all the 100-plus medical specialties practiced in the U.S., the CDC requires only reproductive endocrinologists to report outcomes of their work, and then it's only for one kind of treatment: in vitro fertilization (IVF). Moreover, by the time the data is reported, verified and published, it's three years old with declining usefulness to a savvy shopper of fertility docs.

Where, then, does a patient turn?

The desktop referral

In the old days, the patient turned to her primary care physician, a breed that habitually generated nearly all referrals to specialists. She asked around till she found someone who'd been through similar symptoms previously, and with assertiveness and luck, found a family and/or friend recommendation.

All that was BI: before the Internet. Now many roads to new doctors lead through Web searches. Eight million Americans go online daily to research health information – about 100 every second of every hour of the year. Most begin by thoroughly researching their symptoms, diagnosis and possible treatments. Only then do they look for doctors.

Then they use terms such as "Minneapolis cancer doctors" and "Dallas orthopedic surgeons" and "Oregon hip replacements." This kind of effort narrows the field by simply identifying nearby physician candidates for a patient in need. Inevitably, however, the patient goes to the next question, "Just how good are any of these physicians I've found?"

Increasingly, this prospective patient isn't asking another doctor or even a friend or a family member for the answer to this question. She's asking a stranger. Or, rather, she's asking as many strangers as possible, just like she asks strangers about other goods and services.

In my firm's observations, the social medium with the biggest potential impact on physicians today is rate-your-doctor websites. They're everywhere – from Yelp.com to RateMDs.com to HealthGrades.com – swelling in visits and consumer reviews at an unprecedented rate. And they're having a growing effect on patients' selection of physicians, according to mounting evidence.

If your practice has not had a bad review (or reviews) on a rate-your-doctor website, it's in a small and shrinking minority. Medical practices are increasingly perplexed in how to address online reviews and ratings.

These rate-your-doctor websites may become (or already be) the biggest force in social media for making or breaking a practice. It's not uncommon to meet a newcomer to your city in search of a new primary care physician. Sure, the newcomer is likely to ask around work or the neighborhood for recommendations. But how many stop there? What portion peruses the Web for patient reviews? If moviegoers are reluctant to put down $9 or $10 on a new flick without checking online and newspaper reviews, it's a pretty sure bet that patients increasingly aren't going to place a blind bet on their new doctor.

Here's how a recent conversation went with a co-worker of mine who'd just made an appointment with a new PCP:

"I looked at his online reviews and discovered this doctor had not one but two bad online patient ratings," she related. "One would have been fine, perfectly acceptable. But multiple complaints made me suspect that there was a real problem."

She promptly canceled the appointment and found another PCP with better reviews. While that's one anecdote, there's plenty more evidence that rate-your-doctor websites are as formidable a factor as Facebook or anything else:

1. *A sharp increase in the number of ratings of our client physicians.*

2. *The frequency of practices asking help in dealing with negative reviews.*

3. *Data on visitors to practices' websites.*

On the first point, my firm has been monitoring these sites for quite a while. A year or two ago, our client physicians typically received a trickle of reviews. The trickle has since grown to a steady stream and in some cases a torrent, sometimes because of negative reviews.

On the second point, more and more practices are certain that particular negative reviews are the work of fiercely competitive physicians and/or disgruntled ex-employees – some of whom have gone to work for competitors. Of course, it's often difficult to tell the difference between the reviews of real patients and "flamers" (people who initiate extreme verbal attacks). But some reviews are more overt hoaxes, sufficiently lacking in details and repetitiously vague in their complaints.

Thirdly, a patient on the verge of selecting a physician is more likely to focus on Yelp.com or RateMDs.com reviews after she has visited the practice website. The rate-your-doctor sites usually list so many physicians for each specialty that it's difficult to gauge any individual within the rather vanilla pages of this medium. Most display no photos of the doc (unless the doc pays for the privilege), scant detail on the practice overall, particularly
the more personal look and feel of the practice that can be conveyed through a well executed website.

In short, a visit to a rate-your-doctor site is likely one of the final stops before a patient contacts a practice for an appointment.

Learning from hotels & restaurants

People know how customer-review websites work: anyone can say almost anything – anonymously, of course – about the business being rated. You need only establish a free

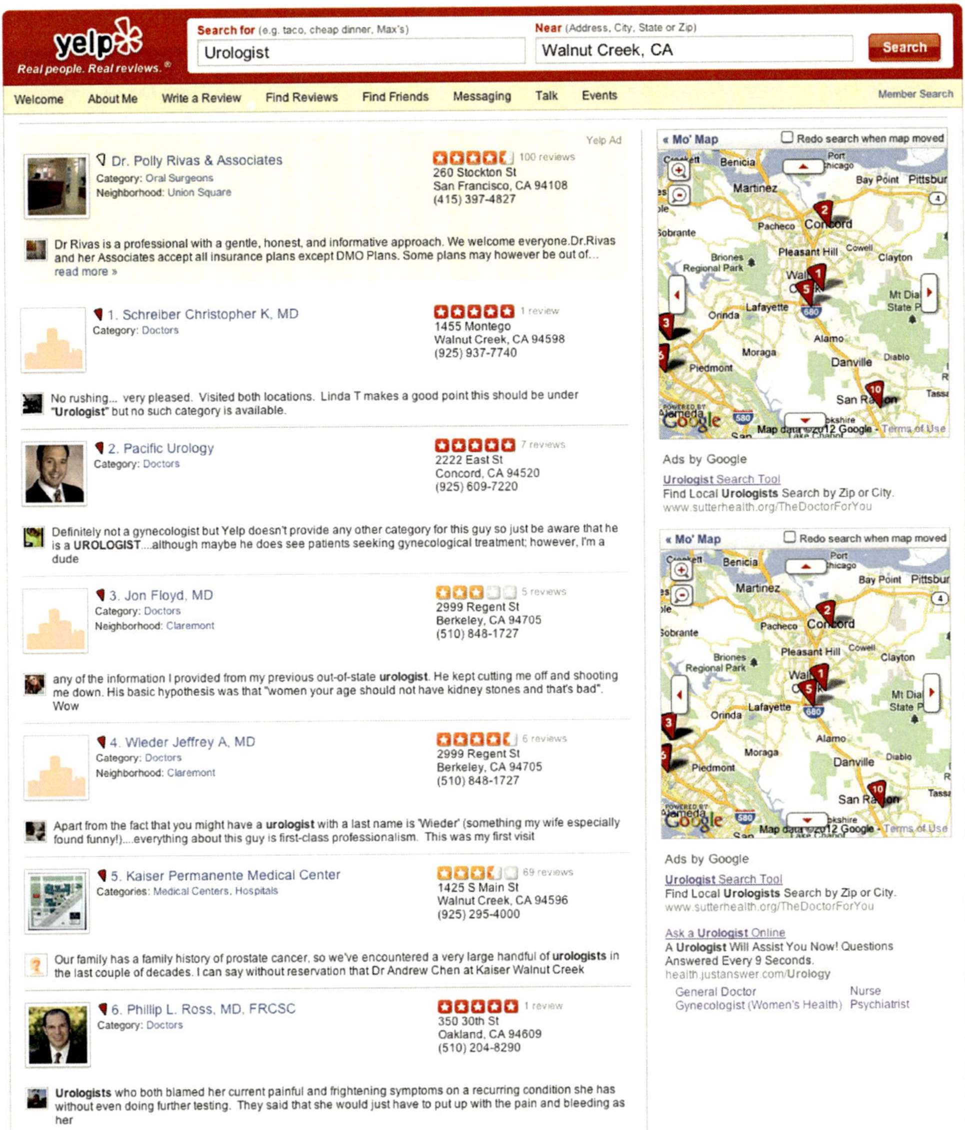

account with one of these sites; then you log in and speak your mind about the business (or doctor) of your choice.

Rate-your-doctor sites require no evidence from any reviewer that she's even met the subject of her critique. Yes, some sites have a few safeguards against flagrant abuses. For example, some sites employ human editors to troll for habitual flamers. In some cases these sites have removed the most hateful comments and banned the commenters.

But these are less-than-perfect safeguards, and the instigator can merely register with the site under a new identity. So is a medical practice helpless? Naturally, a practice cannot control its reviews on rate-your-doctor sites. But a practice can most definitely influence the reviews through a combination of good clinical work, excellent customer service and proactive communications.

Furthermore, in some cases, a practice can address the most stinging reviews directly. Most rate-your-doctor websites allow physicians to establish free personal accounts on the site (if for nothing else than to gather more marketing data).

For these sites, the registered physician often can communicate directly to the complainer and/or comment publicly on the complaint on the same Web page. Sometimes this kind of interaction leads to a happy resolution for all, thereby transforming the complaint into glowing praise for the doctor and the practice.

In the same vein and also the bigger picture, let's not forget that excellent customer service includes excellent customer communications. Part of that service includes giving patients a chance to register their complaints privately and get them addressed – before they feel they have no choice but to squawk on a public website.

With this in mind, patient-satisfaction surveys are a must. I believe in incorporating them into the practice's website and telling every patient about them at the practice's

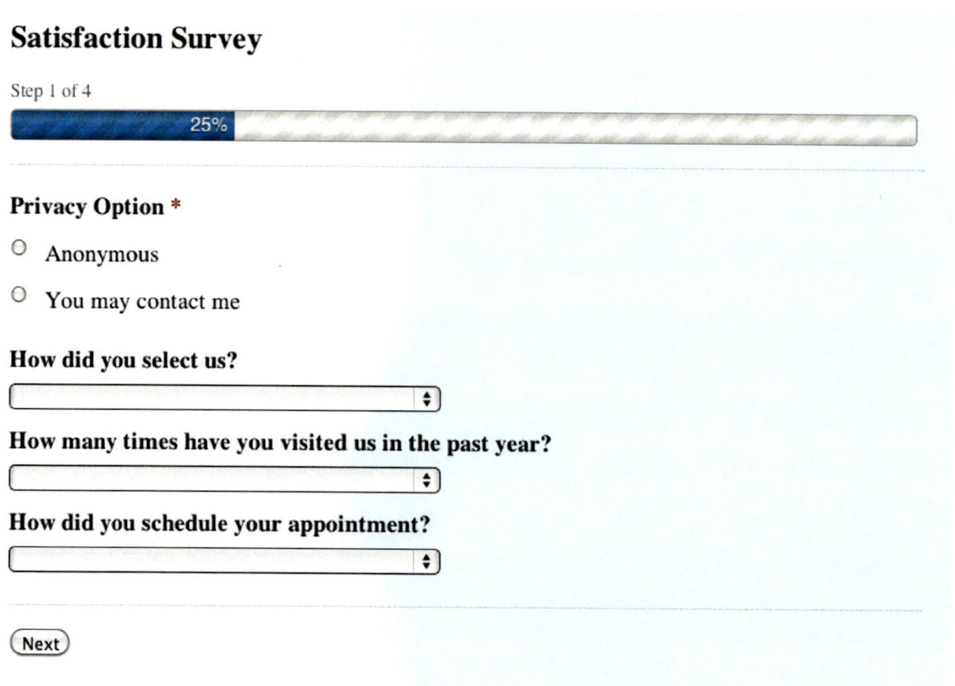

checkout station.

By tackling positive and negative reviews head on, you can make rate-your-doctor websites work in your favor. As with all other forms of social media, the complexities of review websites boil down to communication, and the importance of participating in the online conversation.

Postscript

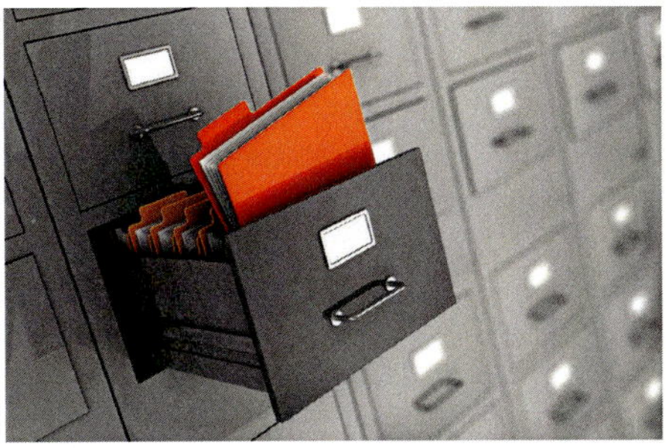

Why bother?

The business case for investing resources

Many years ago, when I made a conscious decision to shift my career focus from general marketing to medical marketing, I did so with full awareness of certain consequences. Physicians traditionally have not only dismissed marketing as unnecessary for their profession; they've also typically disdained it as dishonest and demeaning.

Such views are changing, although there are still plenty of residual effects from the old-fashioned mind-set. Physicians and medical practices rarely have had to pay for marketing in the past – until recent changes in pharmaceutical regulations, most health care marketing was done by pharmaceutical companies, medical device manufacturers and hospitals, not by independent medical practices. As a result, marketing is frequently an expense that doctors and practices are not accustomed to. The scale of the costs can be quite frightening.

For many years, I would regularly check data gathered by the U.S. Department of Commerce on the cost of marketing for businesses in every industrial sector, including health care. In virtually every industry, I found the average marketing budget ran from 4 to 7 percent of gross revenues for businesses that wanted to maintain their market share, and up to 15 percent or more for aggressive companies in search of a larger market share. In contrast, it's rare to find a medical practice spending even 2 percent of collected revenues on finding and recruiting new patients.

For many, however, a modest investment of that scope can have significant effects. When a practice hires our firm to help grow patient volume, our goal is to increase new-patient visits by 10 to 30 percent in the first 12 months. If we've screened each prospective client carefully and the practice is well managed – that is, can deliver excellent clinical care, outstanding customer service and prompt response to new-patient inquiries

– we succeed.

For most multi-physician practices, an increase of 10 to 30 percent in new-patient visits usually results in an annual revenue growth in the six figures, if not seven (for larger practices). This increase in revenue is comparable to adding two nurses to a clinic staff. Somehow, marketing doesn't seem like such a big expense when it's viewed in this context.

Despite such attractive math, there are caveats galore in this game of investing in Internet-driven marketing. For the most skeptical of doubters, I leave you with three factors to keep front of mind when weighing the risks and benefits.

1. The online store principle

Combined with social media and online public relations programs, an effectively managed website (i.e., one that is constantly fed and updated with patient-centric information) acts as a practice's virtual store. You can't examine and treat patients through a website (although that day may be coming), but you sure as heck can start the conversation that leads to patient recruitment. Website activity is stunningly easy to measure and monitor, thanks to free and low-cost software called website analytics.

A practice with a patient-oriented website (including plenty of relevant health information and ways to interact online with the practice) will almost always see increases in the number of visits to the website, more time spent on the site by each visitor, and more pages viewed. As you'd expect, the more time a prospective patient spends in a store – in this case, a thoroughly useful health-resource website – the more likely s/he will make a purchase.

2. Directly measurable effects

Evidence of the above principle can be gathered through other website tools, notably forms for visitors to request information and appointments, as well as call-tracking systems. With these tools, a practice can measure precisely how many visitors contact the practice either online or by phone to request more information or make an appointment.

There are plenty of other ways to measure impact. Again in my firm, we track more than 100 metrics every month as indicators of success in reaching and affecting the target audience. We can interpret much from these metrics, with varying degrees of certainty, that the efforts are indeed having impacts – which leads us to the final point, a reality that businesses of virtually every kind and size must live with.

3. Dotted-line effects

The hardest aspect to accept about marketing is that it is a correlative endeavor and not causative. To be sure, medicine has its own parallels. For example, earlier we discussed how we may know the aggregated five-year survival rate after a certain kind of cancer treatment, based on studies and trials of thousands of patients. But will a single patient be alive five years after the treatment – yes or no? And how does anyone reduce his odds of getting cancer in the first place?

Marketing, with the end goal of changing human behavior, is just as tough to predict and attribute cause and effect in individual cases. However, we marketers can say this with confidence, much as oncologists advise patients with cancer: Your chances of survival are diminished if you pursue none of the treatments and good health habits associated with success.

In short, doing things the old way is less and less of an option for medical practices. To the contrary, empirical evidence and statistical indicators reveal that doing things the new way brings success in the vast majority of cases, although we still may not know if it's from three workouts a week or five (metaphorically speaking).

In the end, I say simply: Eat your vegetables, break a sweat daily, and chances are, you'll have a long and prosperous business life.

42823609R00074

Made in the USA
Middletown, DE
22 April 2017